Y0-BSM-700

Yoga
for
Athletics

Yoga for Athletics

Monica Lind Hathaway
Harmon Hathaway
with Peter Livingston

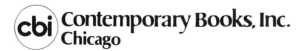
Contemporary Books, Inc.
Chicago

Library of Congress Cataloging in Publication Data

Hathaway, Harmon.
  Yoga for athletics.

  Includes index.
  1. Exercise.   2. Sports.   3. Yoga, Hatha.
4.   Physical fitness.   I. Hathaway, Monica Lind,
joint author.   II. Livingston, Peter, joint author.
III. Title.
GV481.H26   1978   613.7'1   78-57468
ISBN 0-8092-7561-9
ISBN 0-8092-7560-0 pbk.

Photography by Harmon Hathaway, Lori Walsh, and Jeff Laudin

Copyright © 1978 by Monica Lind Hathaway and Harmon Hathaway
All rights reserved
Published by Contemporary Books, Inc.
180 North Michigan Avenue, Chicago, Illinois 60601
Manufactured in the United States of America
Library of Congress Catalog Card Number: 78-75468
International Standard Book Number: 0-8092-7561-9 (cloth)
                                    0-8092-7560-0 (paper)
Published simultaneously in Canada by
Beaverbooks
953 Dillingham Road
Pickering, Ontario L1W 1Z7
Canada

This book is dedicated to the yogic masters of all time who managed to achieve liberation from the sources of trouble.

Accuracy is the winner of the game. Accuracy can be known, but there is no owner of the accuracy.
—*Jim Thorpe*

Don't tell me why I should go beyond this state of suffering I find myself in. . . . I already know why. . . . Tell me how.
—*Tibetan saying*

Contents

Acknowledgments

We would like to thank the following for their generous assistance and support: Bob Reese, N.Y. Jets trainer; David Knight, N.Y. Jets; Dr. Joan Kingsley, director, physical education, Oneonta State University College of New York (S.U.C.O.); Ms. Lee Abbot, swimming coach, S.U.C.O.; Mr. Richard Miller, executive director, Y.M.C.A.; Mr. Garth Stam, soccer coach, S.U.C.O.; Carl J. Delberta, president, Oneonta Boys Club; Don Kelly, coach, Delaware Academy, Delhi; Jack Walsh, all-American diver; Walter Peters, photographer; and our students, especially Cindy Southmayd, Dorothy Kochiras, Carol Stenz, Anne Joelle, Jody Sherman, Augustus Lightheart, David Grossman, Geronimo Sands, Lori Walsh, Jeff Laudin, Steve Stepka, Carolyn June, Isabelle Myre, Charles Biname, Lori Belilove, Michael Karlovich, Judy Maras, Bruce Lano, Alice Rienzie, and Norman Lee for their assistance in putting this book together.

Introduction

Foundation yoga

This book was written for one purpose—to improve dramatically your performance in sports. The techniques and movements we use are probably unlike any you have experienced or read about. In a very quiet way they are revolutionary, for this yoga is neither an end in itself nor a system simply to relieve tension. It is a formula for an entirely new way of moving. Foundation Yoga is built on ancient principles but has been developed specifically to be used by athletes in order to achieve the yogic ideal of a flexible, tuned, and balanced body where motion is efficient, precise, effective, and comfortable—like the quick jump of a cat or the balanced swing of a monkey.

One of the few Western athletes who has this pure balanced quality is Pelé, the internationally famous and near legendary soccer champion. Nimble and quick, he masters the playing field with an effortless grace and precision. Never is the movement forced or strained. "My friend," Pelé said recently in an interview, "I do nothing; I simply let the body move."

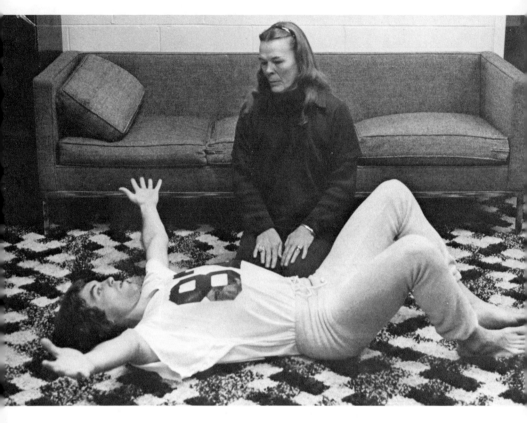

David Knight of the New York Jets practices yogic breathing under the supervision of author Monica Lind Hathaway.

Pelé's remarkable movement on the field demonstrates a profound yogic truth: The human body has an intelligence and balance of its own, and, when it is not interfered with, will perform with natural momentum and precision—as will any animal's. All we need to do is turn the body over to itself, let go of our pictures of how the body should move and should be trained, and simply allow it to be. If this were as easy to do as it is to say, there would be many more star players, far fewer injuries, and no need for a book like ours.

What makes a great athlete?

This question has puzzled athletes, coaches, and trainers for some time, but the best answer seems to be that it's a lot of "little things." The great athlete, the "natural," is not necessarily the strongest, biggest, or best motivated or conditioned, but he or she is invariably loose, relaxed, and nimble—qualities we are quick to admire but often are at a loss to acquire or teach. The star player himself rarely knows how he or she "does it."

Our own natural ability is suppressed by the way we think about and treat the body. We work out with the idea of conditioning, learning, and training rather than opening, loosening, and discovering. We exercise in straight lines and at sharp angles and rarely experience the full, fleshy quality of the body and the open space around it. We admire muscles of "steel" and work to build them while we ignore the line and movement of flesh and bone. And when we do "relax," we usually fall into a limp collapse instead of releasing the tensions that consume our energy. These conditions are so habitual and pervasive that we need a totally new approach to the body if we are to uncover our natural ability.

Freeing the body

Foundation Yoga releases tensions and helps restore the body to a state of greater flexibility and strength where natural movement occurs spontaneously. Most of our exercises are designed to create *trembling* and *shaking* in tense muscles, releasing muscular knots and leaving the body with a softer, fuller, more flexible feeling. Unlike regular stretching exercises, there is no danger of muscular damage or of a muscle "snapping back" and having to be restretched. Our exercises may seem more time-consuming than regular stretching exercises, but in the long run they are actually more efficient: The results are deeper and longer lasting. As you release tight muscles you will also be working to realign your posture to a natural position. In

Foundation Yoga you destroy old habits at the same time you reestablish natural movement.

In this work, *being fully aware* of the movement in an exercise is as important as performing it. When you begin to work with an exercise, we want you consciously to intend each movement, following the directions exactly. For example, we often suggest that you lift your *foot* off the ground. This is altogether different from suggesting you lift your *leg* off the ground, although, to someone watching, the two different ways of lifting might appear identical. The real difference is not just in your head; it involves the muscles you use. You are likely to use less energy and muscle when you intend to lift the foot than when you intend to lift the leg. It is a fact that, when walking, most people pull their legs up into the hips and actually shorten the arc of their stride. This habit leads to tight muscles in the stomach and groin. By simply learning how to lift from the foot, you can conserve a tremendous amount of energy and avoid unnecessary tension.

We want you to *start* each exercise by following the directions exactly, but we also want you to let the body play with the exercise once the shaking and trembling begin. Don't try to control the body, and don't become concerned if the shaking becomes very active or you feel like letting out any sounds. Use the exercises as a starting point, and then go with the spontaneity of the body. The trembling and shaking will cease when you stop the exercise.

The amazing basics

The first three chapters on yogic breathing and balance are very important. Work with these chapters first, before you read up on your sport. Once you have learned to breathe fully and move with yogic alignment, you are well on your way to experiencing a nimble, natural movement in your game, whether that means hitting a ball over a net or blocking an opponent on the football field. So please, resist the temptation to try immediately to improve your game. First discover how to open and relax the body, and then read about your sport. The improvement will occur naturally.

To bring greater flexibility to specific areas in the body, study your skeleton in chapter 2 and work with the releasing exercises in chapter 5; these exercises will bring greater freedom of movement and are highly recommended to speed up recovery after an injury.

It works

For many years we were reluctant to publish these exercises: many of them appear so simple that we were afraid that, without our presence, people would not practice for long enough periods of time. But the athletes we've been working with convinced us that anyone who was serious about improving his or her game would give the exercises a fair chance. The results can be remarkable after only one session, if you stay with the exercise long enough to bring about a good period of trembling and shaking. Twenty minutes of shaking is the recommended minimum for even the simplest movement, but 30 minutes to a full hour is preferred.

We are interested in your progress. If you have any questions, problems, or suggestions please write us at our center in upstate New York. We will be more than happy to answer any questions you might have.

Monica Lind Hathaway and Harmon Hathaway
Foundation for the Study of America Yoga
Bovina Center, New York 13740

1

Yogic breathing for the athlete

The way you breathe directly determines the way you experience life. At one end of the spectrum we have no breathing and death; at the other, full yogic breathing, which allows us to experience tremendous vitality. Most of us find ourselves somewhere in the middle—technically alive and functioning but performing at levels far beneath what is possible. The yogis have known for a long time that the more fully we breathe, the better we live, perform, and solve problems, from mental puzzles to moves on the playing field.

Athletes who take sports seriously and who concentrate on getting stronger tend to breathe shallowly; they have lost touch with an immediate, alive, sensual sense of the body. The body becomes a machine to be conditioned and controlled instead of a spontaneous, three-dimensional expression of the self. These athletes pay a heavy price. They may be strong, but they are likely to become stiff. Certainly they tire (and retire) and suffer injury much more readily than they should.

What is the difference between a great player and a competent one? Most coaches and pros will agree it is not a matter of "inborn" talent. Somehow the star players have "lucked in" to the proper way to use the body, yet they themselves usually can't explain how they do it. We are all potential "naturals"; we only have to learn how to come in contact with our natural ability. Through the yogic approach to breath and posture covered in these first two chapters, you will release your natural ability. You don't have to *try* so much as you need to be open and aware.

Right now, as you are reading this book, you are probably breathing incorrectly. Why do we suspect this? Because almost everyone we have worked with, including the pros, has never been made aware of proper breathing or been coached in the proper techniques. Through awareness you will discover how you breathe and what you may be doing right or wrong. Then, with a few simple directions and some practice, you will discover how to breathe fully; in time, full yogic breathing will become natural.

Yogic breathing is a cornerstone in Foundation Yoga. If you were to learn nothing else from this book, the yogic breathing technique alone would increase your vitality and improve your precision and endurance in sports. As you read, study the photographs and diagrams carefully and relate them to your own body. The natural athlete in you is waiting to break out and perform. Yogic breathing will help open the door.

How you breathe

The fundamental breathing muscle is the diaphragm, a giant, dome-shaped, platform-like structure horizontally bisecting the body beneath the lungs and heart. In the front, the highest part of the diaphragm connects just behind the bottom of the sternum (breastbone). It attaches in back directly behind the front connection. From these central points the diaphragm flows inward and slightly downward in all directions, connecting at the lower area of the rib cage onto and between the four pairs of flexible ribs.

Place your hands on your lower rib cage at the area of the flexible ribs. Now slowly inhale, taking a breath in through the

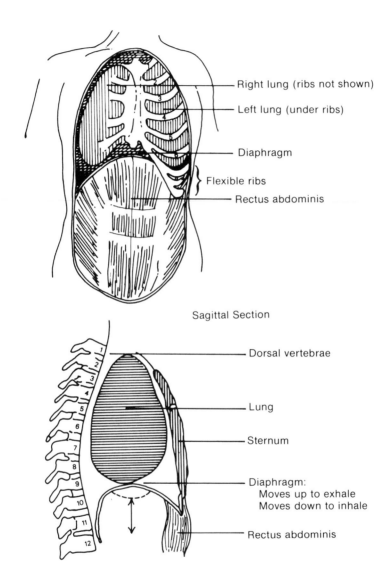

Right lung (ribs not shown)

Left lung (under ribs)

Diaphragm

Flexible ribs

Rectus abdominis

Sagittal Section

Dorsal vertebrae

Lung

Sternum

Diaphragm:
Moves up to exhale
Moves down to inhale

Rectus abdominis

1.1. The diaphragm, front and side views: The diaphragm moves up on the exhale, down on the inhale.

nostrils. Feel these ribs expand in your hands. Now slowly exhale and let the breath rise and go out through the nostrils; feel your ribs contract. Be sure you are taking the breath in through the nostrils and allowing the lungs to fill completely.

The idea of filling the lungs often leads people to try pulling or snorting air upward into the nostrils, which can lead to a blocked, stuffy feeling where the breathing sounds like sniffing. The false inhale tenses the body and produces a rigid feeling, particularly in the lower jaw, neck, and head. Contrary to popular belief, the air holes are not way back in the upper section of the nose but are directly behind the nostrils and only slightly upward. Continue to inhale and exhale slowly, with your hands on your flexible ribs, until you feel comfortable with the in-and-out action of the rib cage.

Now place the thumb of one hand on the point where the diaphragm connects to the bottom of the sternum and the fingers of the other hand on the collarbone.

1.2. With hands on your flexible ribs, you should feel an expansion on the inhale and a contraction on the exhale. The rib cage should not move up or down.

1.3. Neither the collarbone nor the sternum should drop on the exhale. If you feel them moving downward, you are *deflating*, not exhaling.

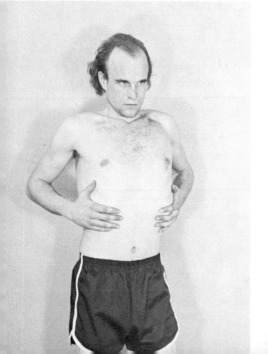

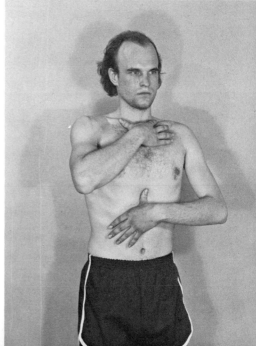

Again, slowly inhale, taking a full breath in through the nostrils. Fill the abdomen and the entire chest cavity. Slowly exhale, letting most of the breath out through the nostrils but keeping some breath in the upper chest cavity. If you experience a downward motion at the sternum or a collapse at the collarbone, you are letting out too much air and are *deflating*; you are not exhaling. Every organ has its own internal space. Deflation causes the rib cage to collapse and the internal organs to become crowded and squashed. In the true exhale, the upper rib cage maintains some air; in deflation the entire rib cage collapses.

If you look at illustrations 1.4 and 1.5 you can see the difference between a true exhale and deflation. As you can see, deflation is a falling and collapsing motion, whereas the true exhale sustains the position of the upper rib cage. In deflation there is no opportunity for the body to utilize the oxygen properly: the falling motion of the rib cage inhibits the interior space of the body and throws the posture off. Breathe as fully as you can, making sure you are exhaling and not deflating.

The simple ability to inhale fully and exhale properly is fundamental to yoga and is essential for good health and athletic

1.4, 1.5. The difference between a true exhale (left) and mere deflation. Notice how proper breathing naturally improves the posture.

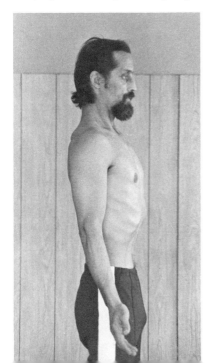
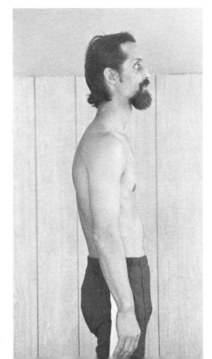

endurance. Once these motions become comfortable, go on to the next section, where you will learn how to expand your breathing capacity and energize your body with breath. A minimum of 20 minutes is recommended to spend on each exercise.

The storage breath and pant

The lungs are the fuel tank of your body. Although they have a potential to store two quarts of air, most of our lungs use only about half that storage capacity. Consequently, we run out of breath much more quickly than we should, and our performance

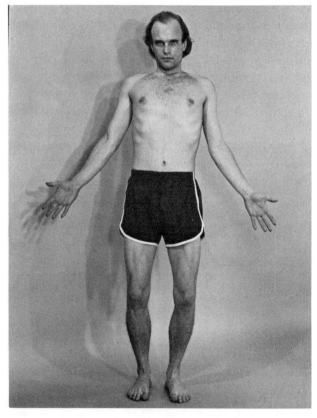

1.6. Storage breath and pant. Lift rib cage with the storage breath and let the pelvis relax and drop. Feel the spine stretch up and down. Open your mouth and pant rapidly.

suffers. The exercises in this section are designed to expand your storage capacity gradually to its full potential.

Stand with your feet pointed straight ahead and allow the weight of your body to radiate down the outside of the feet, through the heel and into the ground. Relax the knees and bend them slightly, as in illustration 1.6.

Now take a full deep breath that lifts the rib cage up off the hip girdle. Allow the collarbone to rise upward with the breath. It's all right if your shoulders rise up toward your ears, so long as your shoulder blades don't pull together or become tense. This first full, deep breath is called a *storage breath*; the idea is to maintain it as you breathe. As the breath lifts the rib cage up off the hip girdle, feel the weight of the hip girdle fall down toward the heels and into the ground. This should give you an expanded sensation of space in the abdomen; it will naturally stretch the spine in two directions, down toward the floor and up into the space above your head. The full breath, lifted rib cage, and dropped pelvis will help to loosen and eventually to eliminate muscle tension that holds the spine in an exaggerated curve (which in extreme cases is called *swayback* or *curvature of the spine*).

When you exhale, allow the breath to flow out from the abdomen, but maintain the storage breath in the upper chest cavity. Now take in another, smaller breath and exhale it. Maintain your storage breath and inhale and exhale quickly through the mouth with a rapid panting rhythm. Check frequently to make sure you have not lost your storage breath.

As you pant, notice that your flexible ribs move in and out at the sides of the body and that there is a similar motion in the space between the ribs. If this does not seem to be happening, it means that your panting is not full enough. Slow down and take deeper pants. If necessary, keep your hands on your rib cage until you are certain your body has accepted the pattern. Do this panting with full storage breath for as long as possible. If your mouth becomes dry, breathe through your nostrils for a while and then return to the mouth. As you continue the pant, you may notice slight twinges of pain in the back or chest. This is a good sign, indicating that the breath is expanding into areas that formerly had been bound with muscle tension. If the pain increases, resist the temptation to stop, but slow down and direct the breath into the painful area. This helps to decrease the pain. Continue to work with the breath, and trust the natural intelligence of your body to use it.

If you have never done deep breathing before, your brain cells will be receiving more oxygen than they are used to; this foreign feeling may generate fear and dizziness. Do not identify with these feelings or any faintness that might accompany them. Just continue to pant, and resist the natural urge to slow down or stop in order to avoid any unpleasantness. You must go through these sensations in order to expand your breathing capacity and arrive at a more vital level of being.

Yogic breathing

The previous exercises were designed to correct your breathing pattern and to expand your breath capacity. Now you are ready to learn the full yogic breathing that should be used at all times. Yogic breathing will bring vitality and a feeling of warmth and fullness throughout the body.

Preliminary exercise

Place a mat or blanket on the floor and lie down on your back. Place your arms slightly away from the torso, palms up. Rest the head at the point just above where the skull sits on the spinal column. Drop your chin down toward your collarbone (illustration 1.7).

Take in a full storage breath and fill the entire rib cage and lower abdomen area, allowing the collarbone to rise up toward the dropped chin. Allow the shoulders to rise up toward the ears. Exhale through the nose about one-quarter of the air you inhaled while you maintain the storage breath. Inhale again, allowing the lower abdomen to expand as fully as possible; as you inhale, let the action of the breath become so full that you

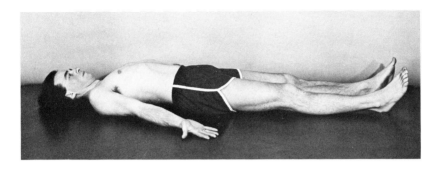

1.7. Full yogic breathing. Lie comfortably on your back, palms up, and begin to fill the abdomen and chest cavity with breath.

experience an expansion throughout the entire chest cavity—up through the back of the neck, through the shoulders, into the head, arms, and hands, and down through the lower torso, through the groin and into the legs and feet. If the body feels tingly and trembles or starts to twitch or stretch, allow these actions to occur. Just continue to bring in as much air on the inhale while you release only one-quarter on the exhale.

Full yogic breathing

Lie down as in the previous exercise and take a full storage breath. Exhale through your nose, letting out as much air as you can *without losing your storage breath*. Breathe in and out slowly and be sure the collarbone does not drop on the exhale. Continue breathing with the idea of allowing the breath to fill the whole body. Be aware that the energy field around the body extends beyond the skin, and imagine the breath expanding out into the space around your body. Do full breathing with the idea of giving the breath to the body to utilize however it wishes. Trust the intelligence of the body to release whatever hidden tensions you have unconsciously harbored, and to fill out and expand any muscle or skeletal collapses that have occurred. As you do this breathing for longer periods of time, you will notice increasing relaxation.

This exercise should also be practiced while standing in the

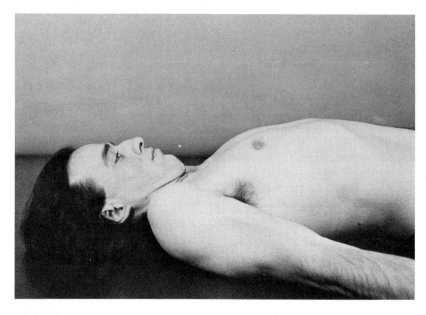

1.8. Full yogic breathing. Expand the entire rib cage with air. Drop chin to the collarbone and allow shoulders to rise up toward the ears as you exhale as deeply as possible.

1.9. Sounding out. Check with your hands to make sure air is emptying completely from the abdomen but remains in the upper rib cage. Open the mouth wide to allow the *ah* sound to flow out.

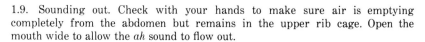

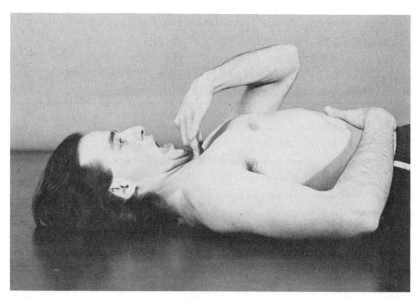

fundamental yogic stance, which is described in the next chapter. Ideally, full yogic breathing should be occurring at all times.

Sounding out

Many people who have successfully learned yogic breathing lose it when they start to speak. The following exercise is designed to enable you to be conscious of yogic breathing while talking.

Lie down on your back, arms out, palms up. Take seven full breaths in and out; on the eighth, exhale slowly, whispering a pure *ah* sound (not *eh* or *uh*). Experiment until you find a comfortable tone. Keep your mouth open, with the jaw dropped all the way down, until the breath from the abdomen is completely expelled. Check to make sure you have not lost your storage breath. You may want to place one hand on your collarbone and the other on your abdomen to make sure the air is releasing completely from the abdomen as you whisper the *ah*, but remaining in the upper rib cage.

The *ah* sound should fill the whole mouth and resonate through the throat. Whisper it 10 times, and then raise the volume to just over a whisper and sound out for another 10 breaths.

Continue to take the volume of the *ah* sound up in small increments, and maintain each volume for 10 exhales until you are at the loudest volume you can produce without strain. Now reverse the process and gradually lower the volume in steps maintaining each level for a full 10 exhales.

Let the sound of *ah* fill the room without evaluating the quality of the sound. Simply let it occur. Throughout the exercise, be sure the sound is pouring out from the full, open inside of the mouth and throat and that you are not trapping it in the nose or teeth.

After you have gotten comfortable with the varying intensities of *ah*, experiment with *ha!* The *ha*, unlike the *ah*, should come forth in a single, powerful burst on a rapid exhale. Place your palms on your abdomen and feel the upward movement of the breath as you let out a powerful *ha!* Now experiment with *ho* and *ha, ha, ha, ha, ho.*

As you practice these exercises, you may experiment with new sounds or even words and sentences. The idea is to get the sensation of the sound riding on the breath so that, when you speak, your words flow outward with the breath and are not pushed out, interrupting the natural rhythm of breathing.

By doing the various exercises in this chapter, your breathing muscles will gradually become freed and tuned to their natural position. Yogic breathing soon will occur without effort or attention. Once this occurs, your body will be much better prepared to supply itself with the extra oxygen and energy it needs for strenuous activity. In the meantime, check your breathing regularly to be sure you have a storage breath and are breathing fully.

2

Yogic flexibility for the athlete

The skeleton

We have found that surprisingly few athletes can visualize how their own skeletons are constructed, the exact location of each joint, and what range of movement is possible at each joint. This lack of accurate knowledge tends to cause undue muscular tension, which inhibits flexibility and balance in performance. Thus, this understanding is essential for advanced yogic practices. In this chapter you will have a chance to experience your skeleton, joint by joint. As you come to know your body better, it will become increasingly clear which areas need the most release and relaxation. These areas can then be worked with the specific exercises in chapter 5.

As you work with the simple movements in this chapter, don't force the joint action by straining muscles. Leave the muscles as relaxed and fleshy-feeling as possible. Note that the movement originates with your *intention* and not in the joint or muscle itself. Moving with this knowledge leaves the body space open to knowing directly how much energy or force is needed for a

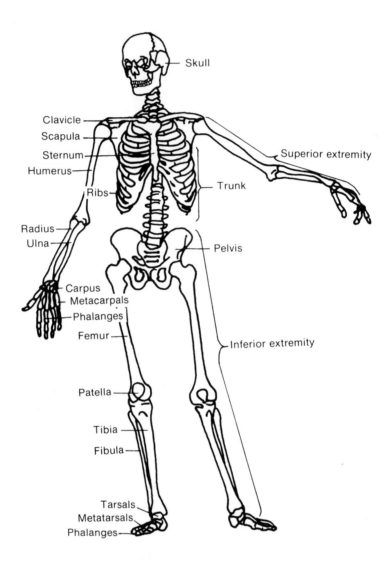

2.1. The skeleton. The athlete must understand its construction in order to experience maximum flexibility and balance.

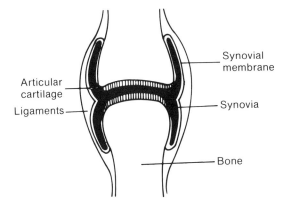

2.2.   The joint. Yogic exercises can help to alleviate muscle tensions, which compress the precious spaces at all joints.

particular movement of play. The body will respond intelligently to a clear intention of what there is to be done.

JOINT

Bones at a joint are tipped with cartilage, a softer-than-bone material that cushions shock. Cartilage is then covered with a thin membrane that encloses a lubricant called synovial fluid. This system of cartilage and synovial fluid prevents wear and tear to the joint.

When your muscles become tense, the space at the joint becomes compressed. In extreme cases of tension and physical activity, the synovial membrane can become damaged and cartilage can wear down. Prolonged muscular tension can cause joint pains of various types and degrees. Thus, it is extremely important to release tension and create a sense of space for movement around every joint in the body.

Each joint allows for the independent movement of a part of the body; yet, because of muscular tension and imbalances in the body, we are seldom able to move one part of the body without another part becoming tense. The legs, for example, have a free swing space of their own, but as we raise one leg, the other tends to react as well. Relaxation through the joints will help to alleviate this condition.

The movements in this chapter are designed so that you can experience and discover the potential motion in the major joints of your body. Don't be surprised if you experience tension around these joints. This is the ordinary condition. Later, in the individual sport sections and especially in the final section, you will find specific exercises designed to release psycho-muscular tension in the joints. But before you begin to make specific corrections in the body, you should know its movement potential. Practice each simple movement in this chapter. They will take you a long way toward the freedom you want to achieve in order to perform at your best.

FOOT

Each foot is composed of 26 bones and 26 joints allowing for tremendous flexibility and movement.

Stand with the weight of your body dropping into the ground through the outsides of the feet and slowly raise your toes and lower them, one at a time, little toes first. Be aware that you can experience the movement of each toe. Do this several times. Now, stand with feet pointing straight forward. Press into the ground with the outside balls of the feet and slowly allow your heels to rise until you are standing on the outside ball and toes. Make sure the weight is dropping into the ground through the outside ball of the foot across to the outside of the big toe and that your knees are relaxed. Now repeat this simple move the *incorrect* (unbalanced) way, by pressing from the inside of the foot. Notice that when you press from the inside, the body is inclined to go forward and the alignment is thrown off.

A properly aligned body begins with the toes and feet. Remember, the proper weight distribution along the outside of the feet is fundamental for correct body alignment.

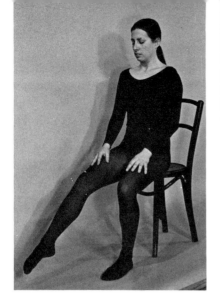
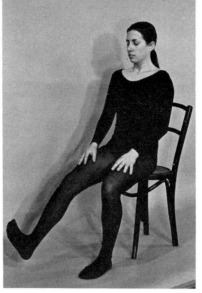

2.3.   Flexing the ankles. First rotate
the foot, from inside to outside.

2.4.   Now flex the foot upward, then
downward, as far as you can.

ANKLE

Most people have an erroneous idea about the actual location of this joint and imagine it to be higher than it actually is. The ankle joint is beneath the two protruding bones (tibia and fibula) at the end of the leg, where they meet two bones in the foot.

Sit down on a chair and raise one foot at a time and rotate the foot toward the outside and then toward the inside so that you feel the full movement in the ankles. Now flex your foot upward toward your shin; then extend your foot down as far as you can.

Simple repetition of these motions will also help return normal movement after an ankle injury.

KNEE

The knee joins the two lower leg bones (fibula and tibia) and the upper leg bone (the femur). Contrary to most people's image, the knee joint is actually below and behind the kneecap.

Stand on your right foot, raise the left foot up toward the buttock and then swing the left foot straight out, as in illustration 2.6.

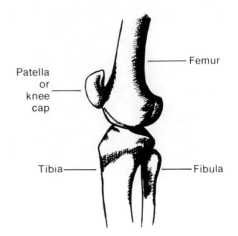

2.5. The knee joint. The
knees should always feel loose,
never locked.

2.6. The knee swing.
Concentrate on the *back* of the
knee joint.

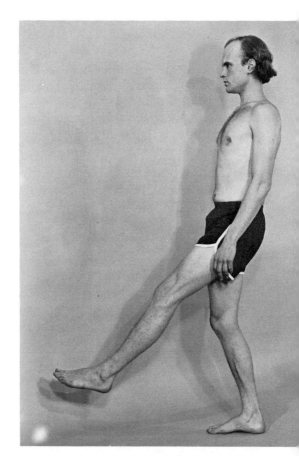

Focus your attention on the back of the knee joint and feel the source of the movement. Now swing in slow motion. Repeat the swing standing on the left foot. One should really get acquainted with the fact that the full, free movement of the knee originates at the back of the joint. Commonly the athlete places the weight of his body on the front part of the knee and thereby puts an undue strain on the joint—and throws the body forward and off balance. The knees should always feel loose and never locked.

Hip joint

If you study the skeleton on page 14 you will notice that the upper leg bone connects to the hip girdle higher than you might have imagined. It is another misconception for people to picture their legs beginning on a line with the crotch. Predictably, this idea inhibits the full swing of the leg.

Stand in the basic stance and bend forward from the hip joint (*not* the waist or crotch), without moving your buttocks backward, as in illustration 2.7. Run your hands along your buttocks and hamstrings and try to let go of any tension so that the muscles feel as soft as possible. Then slowly rise and stand upright. Experiment with this bend several times.

Now place your right hand on your right knee and left hand on your left buttock, as in illustration 2.8.

Shift the weight into your left leg and shift the left buttock out to the side, as far as you can. Bend, and gently stretch in this position. Now reverse the position, shifting your weight into your right leg and moving your right buttock out, as in illustration 2.9. Shift back and forth as you explore the flexibility of this region.

Spine

As you can see from illustration 2.10, the lower back is composed of the coccyx and the sacrum and lumbar portions of the spine. The sacrum and coccyx are fused vertebrae; actual motion in the spine begins at the first joint of the lumbar section

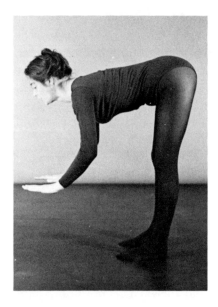

2.7. The hip bend. Bend from the hip joint, not the waist or the crotch.

2.8. With hands in place, shift weight into your left leg and shift the left buttock to the side.

2.9. Now reverse shifting weight into the right leg and buttock.

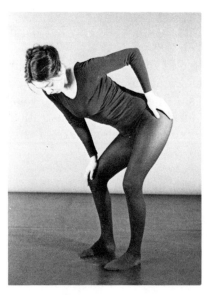

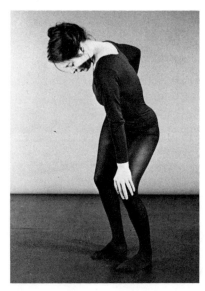

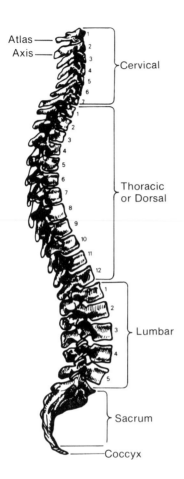

Atlas

Axis

Cervical

Thoracic
or Dorsal

Lumbar

Sacrum

Coccyx

2.10. The spine. Actual
motion begins at the first joint
of the lumbar section.

and continues upward at each vertebra. Experience the flexibility of the lower lumbar region by bending from side to side.

Also try tilting your pelvis forward and backward (like a
belly dancer executing a bump) and swiveling your hips.

There should be about six inches of space in the lumbar
region, from the top of the hip girdle to the lowest rib, and
approximately two to three inches on the sides. If the muscles in
this area are tight, the space may be compacted and should be
opened up.

The upper spine is composed of the 12 dorsal vertebrae to

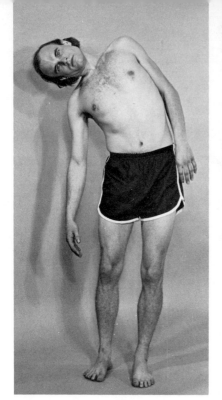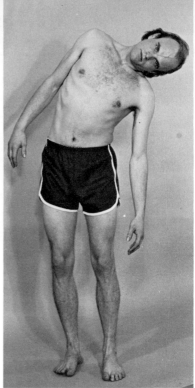

2.11, 2.12. Bend from side to side to experience the flexibility of the spine.

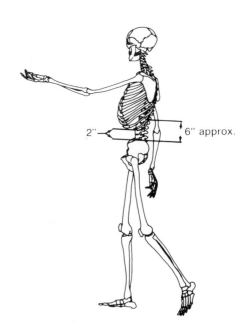

2" ___→   6" approx.

2.13. Space in the body. With
proper breathing, there should
be approximately six inches in
the back between the hip
girdle and ribs, and two to
three inches at the sides.

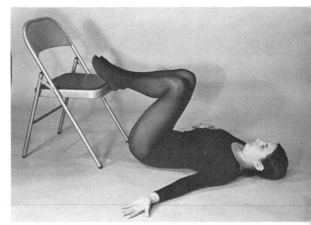

2.14. Spine roll. To experience flexibility of the entire spine, first lie down as shown, feet resting against a chair or a couch.

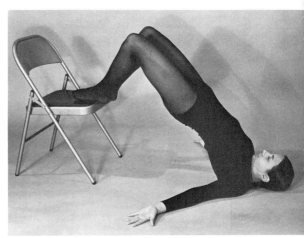

2.15. Now press against the edge and lift the buttocks to form a full arch in the back.

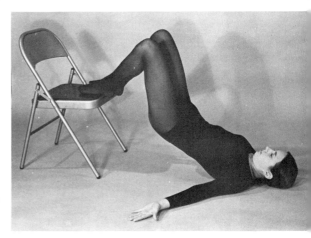

2.16. Then lower the body slowly, vertebra by vertebra, being aware of any tensions.

which the ribs attach, and the seven cervical vertebrae above which complete the spine.

To experience the full flexibility of the entire spine, lie down on your back with your knees bent and your feet resting against the seat of a chair or couch, as shown in illustration 2.14.

Now press against the chair and lift the buttocks off the ground until you feel a full arch in the back. The weight should be falling toward the ground through your neck and shoulders. Slowly lower the body so that your spine touches the ground, vertebra by vertebra.

Repeat this motion, called the *spine roll*, several times and be aware of any tensions that prevent it from being smooth.

SHOULDER GIRDLE AND ARMS

The shoulder girdle is composed of the two collarbones (clavicle), two shoulder blades (scapula) and two upper arm bones (humerus). Remarkably, this interlocking structure has only one skeletal connection with the body, where collarbones join the top of the sternum. The entire girdle has a free-floating nature that allows for tremendous movement and flexibility. If you trace the collarbone out from the sternum, you'll notice that it joins the top of the scapula above the shoulder joint. The humerus joins

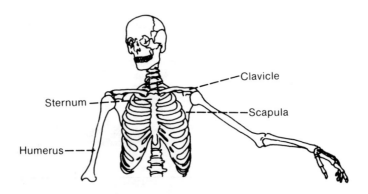

2.17. The shoulder girdle and arms: A free-floating system that allows for tremendous movement and flexibility.

the underside of the scapula to form the shoulder joint. The following movement will allow you to feel the full flexibility of the upper body.

Lift the shoulders up toward the ears and then bring the shoulder blades together, as in illustrations 2.18 and 2.19.

From this position, lower the shoulders and then raise them again. Now open the shoulder blades and bring the shoulders as far forward as possible and lower them, as in 2.20 and 2.21.

Repeat the same sequence of movements with the arms raised straight above the head.

If you're like most people, you'll feel some pain and tension in the shoulders and along the spine. This is an area with tremendous potential flexibility; later in this book you'll find extensive exercises that will help release the muscles which are causing you pain and preventing full movement.

Most people you see suffer from one of two conditions: Either the muscles of the shoulder area are strained away from the spine in a forward hunch, or they are jammed into the spine in a militaristic posture. Both conditions are unnatural and lead to many aches and pains. The following movement is designed to help you arrive at the proper alignment of this area.

Raise your hands straight out to the sides, palms up. Now rotate your arms backward and trace four small circles. Now make four medium-sized circles and finally trace four large circles, bringing your hands all the way down to your sides and all the way up over your head. Illustrations 2.22 through 2.29 demonstrate this step by step.

On the last large circle, let the hands come to rest as far back and down as possible. Now slowly raise the hands, palms up, and keep them behind the ears until they meet over the head, as illustrated by 2.30, 2.31, and 2.32.

Slowly twist the palms outward and continue in slow motion to bring the arms back down to the position you started from, being sure you keep them behind the ears all the way. If you feel a slight tingling sensation in your fingers, it means that nerve connections along the spine have been stimulated.

It is important to understand that the upper arm joint is not at the top of the shoulder but underneath it. You can experience

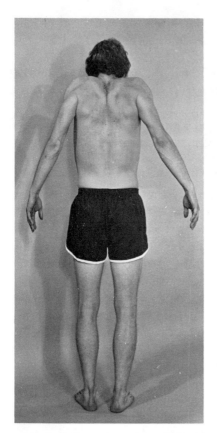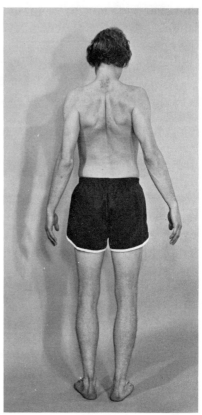

2.18, 2.19.   The shoulder flex. First lift shoulders toward the ears, bringing the shoulder blades together (left). Then, blades still together, lower the shoulder.

this by placing the fingers of the right hand an inch below your left shoulder and swinging the left arm from the joint below. Repeat with the opposite hand and shoulder. See illustration 2.33.

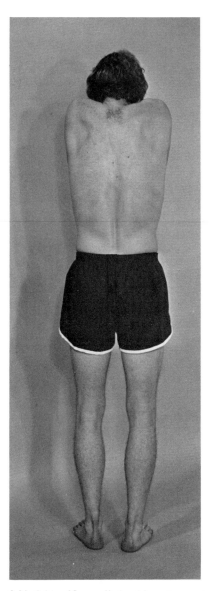 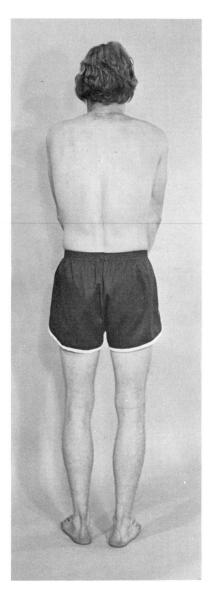

2.20, 2.21. Now roll shoulders forward and up (left). Then lower the shoulders.

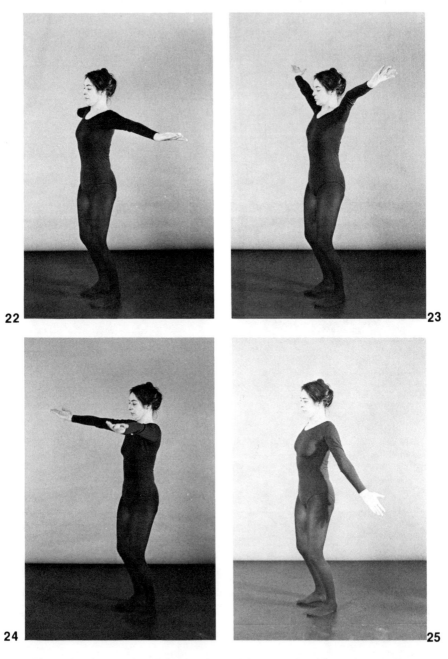

2.22–2.29. Arm rotation. Raise hands straight out to the sides, palms up. Rotate arms backward and trace four small circles. Now make four medium-sized circles and finally trace four large circles, bringing hands all the way down to

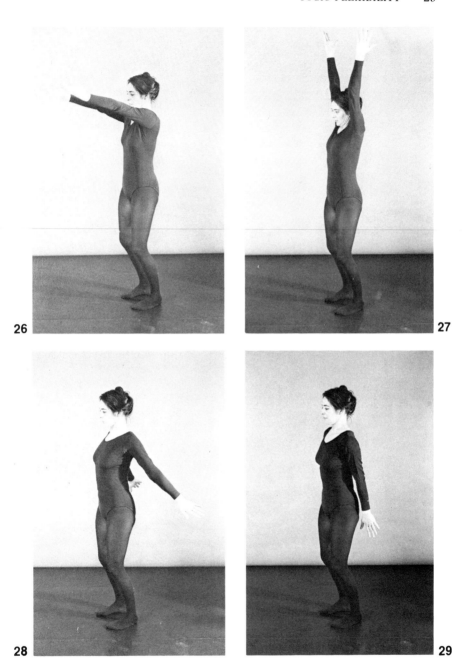

26

27

28

29

your sides and all the way up over your head. After the last large circle, let the
hands come to rest as far back and down as possible.

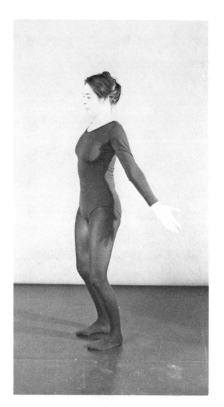

2.30–2.32. Now slowly raise hands, palms up, and keep them behind the ears until they meet over the head. Then slowly twist the palms outward and, keeping them behind the ears all the way, very slowly lower arms to the starting position.

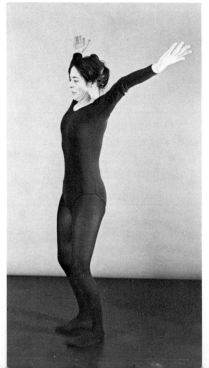

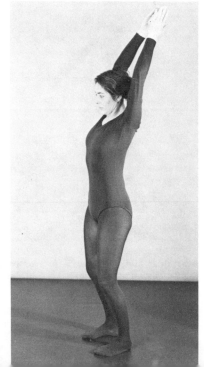

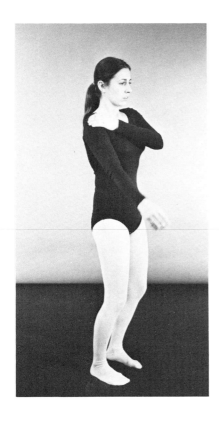

2.33.   Arm joint swing. Feel the location of the upper arm joint by placing the fingers of the right hand one inch below the left shoulder and swinging the left arm.

The elbow is a three-point connection joining the upper arm bone (humerus) with the lower arms bones (radius and ulna). You can experience two types of motion at the elbow: *flexing* and *extending* plus a *rotation* of the lower arm. Experience the rotation by keeping the upper arm still and turning the palm up and down. (Specific exercises for the elbow are in chapter 5.)

The wrist is composed of the two lower arm bones and three bones (carpals) in the hand, which allows for extensive motion. The hand alone has 27 bones and joints, which enable people to perform such incredible feats of flexibility and speed as playing the piano, Spanish castanets, guitar and other string instruments, besides walking and balancing on your hands. Experiment with these types of movement.

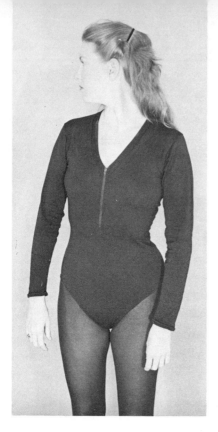

2.34. Head turn. Slowly turn your head right from the axis, until the chin is directly over your shoulder. Repeat in opposite direction.

HEAD AND NECK

Above the 12 dorsal vertebrae are seven cervical vertebrae, which make up the neck. The sixth, the axis, allows the head to rotate from left to right, while the seventh, the atlas, allows the head to move up and down. The combined action of the atlas and axis allows the head to make a smooth, rotary motion.

Most people are inclined to move their heads from the front of the neck and chin, causing protruding vertebrae at the top of the shoulders and tensions that can result in headaches. The following motion is designed to help you feel the proper alignment of the neck and skull.

Take a full storage breath and drop the chin toward the collarbone. Then slowly turn your head right from the back (at the axis), until your chin is directly over your shoulder (illustration 2.34).

Now, slowly turn your head until your chin rests over your

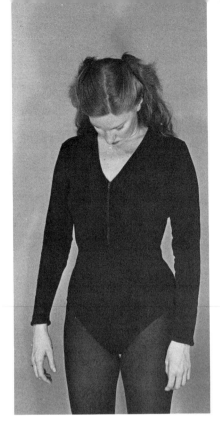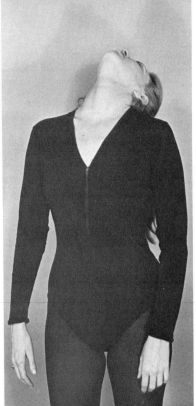

2.35, 2.36. Head drop. Experience the up-and-down motion of the atlas by slowly moving the head as far down as possible (left) and then as far back as possible.

other shoulder. Repeat this slow turning of the head from shoulder to shoulder about 10 times.

Now experience the up-and-down motion of the head (at the atlas) by slowly moving the head as far down as possible and then raising it back as far as possible.

Repeat this 10 times. Now rotate the head in a complete circle. (The atlas and axis work together.) Circle from left to right five times, and then from right to left five times. Be aware of the rotation point at the back of the head.

Each of the movements in this chapter will aid you in experiencing the full use of the principal joints in the body, each of which should be fully experienced and appreciated. (If you wish to explore your anatomical structure further, the classic *Grey's Anatomy* is excellent.)

3

Yogic balance and alignment for the athlete

Body and mind can interfere with one another and deprive us of health and vitality—or they can work together harmoniously. Unfortunately, many people impose an *idea* of how they should look onto their bodies, thus causing bizarre geometries of muscular tension and posture. A typical example is the different way men and women walk. The strong macho stride of the male is as common as the slinky, seductive posture of a female. Both, of course, are unnatural and can eventually cause pain and damage to the body. The male or female body already portrays its natural sexuality, and exaggerated efforts to heighten it, or to change it to match some cultural ideal, only mask the body's real nature.

We are all subject to hopes, fears, and ambitions, but instead of fully experiencing and examining them, we too often subconsciously lock them in our musculature for all the world to see. People who want to get ahead and who are always in a rush go forth in the world with protruding necks and shoulders. They lead with their heads instead of with their feet. The entire torso leans forward, and when they walk rapidly they look as if they are about to fall on their faces. The recent popularity of high-heeled shoes for both sexes heightens this forward lean.

Fear, as common in the Western world as aggression and ambition, can cause the body to become tense and subtly collapsed in a subconscious retreat from the world. Flat feet, crossed legs, and hunched shoulders are all body signs of retreat and anxiety. Our modern environment is so fast-paced and success oriented that it is rare to find anyone without undue muscular tension and postural imbalance. This misuse of energy deprives all of us of vitality and stamina.

These same tensions, which can be seen in virtually everyone to a greater or lesser extent, wreak havoc on the athlete. Ideas about winning and getting ahead worsen the situation, because the body is constantly being "conditioned" from an aggressive point of view. The idea of winning is inherent in every game; it is not something that needs to be concentrated upon. Our awareness should be on the play as it is happening. An open, relaxed body will be best able to master the action as it occurs. A perfect example of this philosophy can be seen in the way Muhammad Ali moved in the ring as heavyweight champion. Unlike most fighters, who crouch and lean forward in pursuit of the attack and the win, Ali's winning stance is open. He dances in the space and actually uses the aggression of his opponent to tire him and throw him off balance.

When an athlete is stiff, anxious, muscle-bound, and collapsed, he loses agility and accuracy, no matter how strong he may be.

The sequence of exercises in this chapter is designed to help the athlete let go of tensions that distort a natural balance and posture. By slowly discovering the natural yogic stance and learning how to walk, jump, and run from it, the athlete will be freed from accumulated tension and poor postural habits. Improved endurance, accuracy, and agility will occur naturally.

Using the full ground

The exercises in Foundation Yoga are deceptively simple, so simple, in fact, that you may be tempted to avoid doing some of them or not doing them for long enough periods of time. Unlike muscle building exercises, where the results of your effort may not be apparent until after weeks or months of practice, the results in Foundation Yoga can be dramatic after only one session—if you practice with full attention for a long enough period of time. If the idea arises that the following exercises are silly and pointless, simply admit your doubts to yourself and continue with the exercise. Let your body play with the movement and enjoy itself.

There is an old saying that you have to be able to crawl before you can walk and walk before you can run. In this exercise you are going to crawl in order to experience the flexibility of your back muscles as you used them as a baby. You are going to get acquainted with the ground through your hands and knees. This exercise is surprisingly effective in freeing up stiff torso muscles—and rigid mental views.

Choose a room with as much uncluttered space as possible, preferably with a well-cushioned rug or mat on the floor. Get down on your hands and knees in the center of the room and drop the lumbar region of your back down toward the belly button area. Relax all your stomach muscles, allowing your stomach weight to fall toward the ground. Your palms, shins, and ankles should be in full contact with the ground if possible. Your shoulders should be relaxed, with your forearms directly in front of your knees. Look straight ahead.

Crawl in a straight line using opposite hand from knee. Crawl to the end of the room and then back again. Do this straight-line crawl four to six times and then crawl in a large circle around the room. Once you have gotten a comfortable feeling with the crawl, play with various speeds and different size circles. Turn around in one spot or move in longer crawl motions. Be sure you are aware of the ground through the parts of your body that touch it. As you play with this exercise, you can come in contact with the adeptness of a baby.

A baby crawls without knowing the word *crawl*. At that stage all of us were free to discover movement rather than imitating the movements of others. Try to remember what you expe-

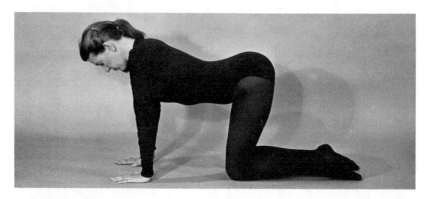

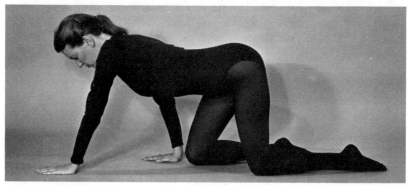

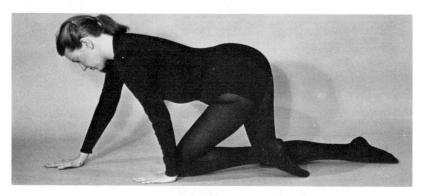

3.1–3.3. The crawl. Start with the stomach completely relaxed and hanging down (top). Move forward slowly, advancing left hand and right knee (center). Continue moving forward, advancing opposite hand and knee simultaneously.

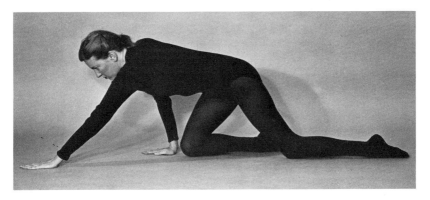

3.4. The cat. Play with the crawl by elongating the movements and slinking along like a cat stalking its prey.

rienced physically as a baby. You may discover you remember emotional responses to your environment rather that true body sensations and experiences. Try to get in touch with the feeling of crawling as a baby, and then experiment and play.

Now come in contact with the lithe, sleek movement of a cat (3.4). Make long, slow reaches with the hands and knees as a cat does when it stalks its prey. Be aware of the length of the spine and move the head in various directions. Get in touch with the length of your arms and legs. Notice areas of tension and try to find movements that help release it.

The cat, like the baby, is nonintellectual master of natural movement. The ability to move naturally is still within you, and these exercises will help you to rediscover it.

Fundamental stance

Every athlete needs a full awareness of the ground and the three-dimensional space surrounding the body. When our posture is misaligned and our muscles are tense, we actually resist gravity and inhibit the free, balanced movement of the body that is so important in athletics. In this exercise you will learn how to let your weight drop into the ground through an aligned skel-

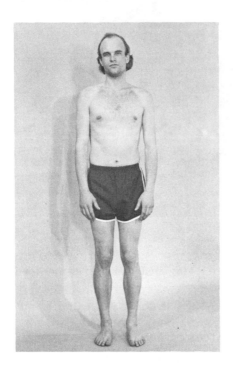

3.5. Body collapse. The whole body, from the ankles to the shoulders, turns *inward*.

eton. The exercise may cause some discomfort as muscles and bones subtly shift position, but the rewards will be well worth the effort. Once you have learned how to stand yogically the transition to walking, running, and participating in sports will develop naturally.

Wear a bathing suit or a leotard or work in the nude in a room with as much open space as possible. Stand with your feet about 6 to 8 inches apart, toes pointing straight ahead. Lift your rib cage up with a full storage breath and practice yogic breathing for a few minutes.

Now look down at your feet, ankles, and knees. If you're like many of the athletes we've worked with, you'll notice an inward collapse beginning with the feet and ankles and continuing all the way up the legs, as in illustration 3.5.

You may also notice that your knees are locked and your thighs are pulled together, your pubic bone has probably been rotated under and up toward the buttocks, causing muscular tension in the lumbar region. What we usually call a *flat foot* or a *fallen arch* is an extreme example of the common tendency for the weight of the body to shift into the insides of the feet and legs. Even if you have a high arch, you may still notice an inward turn at the ankle, knee, and hip joints. The smallest inward turn must be corrected.

Be sure to continue doing deep yogic breathing throughout this exercise. Make sure you point your feet straight ahead and keep them about 6 to 8 inches apart so that they are directly beneath the point where the collarbone joins the shoulder joint. Now, from the bottom of your feet, roll slightly outward so the majority of your weight drops into the ground from just under the outsides of the anklebones and heels.

Allow your feet to feel warm, fleshy, and full. The soles of your feet should feel as sensitive as the palms of your hands. Make sure your toes are relaxed and are pointed straight ahead. Be aware of the fact that the ground supports the entire weight of the body, and be aware of the space around the body. Experience the body's three-dimensional nature. Most of us are so forward-oriented, especially in sports where the opponent or goal is usually in front of us, that we are not aware enough of the

3.6. Fundamental stance. Direct weight to the outsides of the feet. Feel the legs, knees, pelvis, and chest area open. Allow shaking to occur!

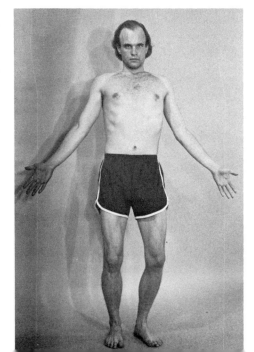

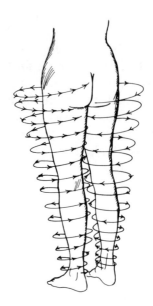

3.7. Outward corkscrews.
This is how you can imagine
energy rising up each leg and
meeting in the back, right
under the tailbone.

open space behind us, above us, and to our sides. Feel the
posture of your body in the open space.

Relax your knee joints and continue to allow your weight to
drop down the outside and back of the body through the point
just under the outside anklebones and the heels.

Now press into the ground through this point and open the
legs by rotating the muscles from the ankle to the hip slightly
outward. Imagine two outward corkscrews of energy rising up
each leg and meeting in the back, right under the tailbone.

Let the knees bend slightly and relax the muscles of the lower
back, allowing the back of the pelvis to drop down toward the
heels. This will cause the genitals and front of the pelvis to
rotate forward. When you find the right position, the opening of
the anus will be relaxed and pointing straight down.

When you first try this stance it may help to reach down, grab
your ankles, and gently twist your legs from the inside to the
outside to get a sense of the outward corkscrews. Slowly guide
your hands upward, twisting outward on your calves, knees, and
thighs.

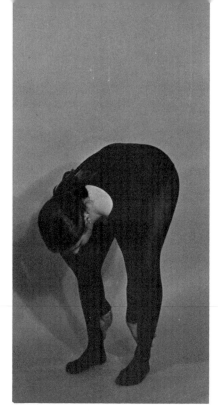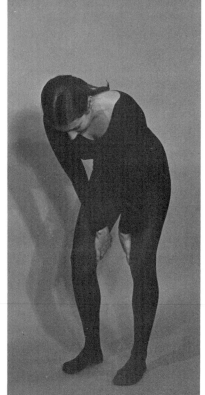

3.8, 3.9. Opening the legs. Reach down, grab ankles, and gently twist up the calves, knees, and thighs, as shown. Then resume the fundamental stance.

Don't actually move the legs; just get the sense of the weight rotating out from the inside of each leg to the outside so that it eventually falls into the ground along the outside edges of the feet, chiefly under the anklebone. Look down and see if you can notice a more open stance in your legs.

Now, bring your chin and neck in so they are not jutting out in front of the body. Let your arms hang comfortably at your sides, but face your palms forward with the fingers separated and stretched outward. Keep your eyes open.

Since you are not used to this position you may experience some discomfort in your joints and muscles or some anxiety at being open and exposed. Continue to breathe fully. If you practice long enough, you will notice a trembling action in the muscles of the legs and possibly in the back, shoulders, and arms. Allow this shaking to occur. This is a sign that the muscles, which have been maintaining a poor posture, are releasing. As they release, the stance will become easier.

If, at the end of 10 minutes, shaking or trembling do not occur, do 10 yogic knee bends. Go straight down, slowly pushing

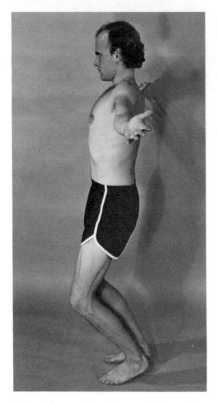
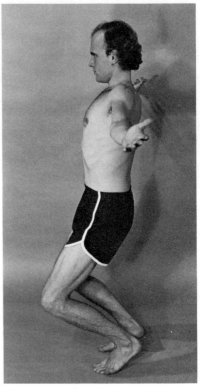

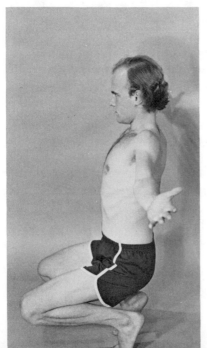

3.10–3.12. The yogic knee bend. With arms out and palms up, go straight down, pushing down the ground with the outside toes. Keep back straight at all times. Even as the heels come off the ground, the weight should still radiate down the back of the body. Keep the breath full.

the ground down with the outside toes as you keep your weight radiating along the back and outside lines of the body into the heels. Keep your back straight throughout the bend. Even as the heels come off the ground, the weight should still be radiating down the back of the body. When rising, push the ground down with the outside toes and allow the heels to go down as soon as possible. Get the idea of a slight downward pressure just above the kneecap. Try to forget the way you are used to doing knee bends and follow precisely the preceding yogic instructions. Move slowly and with full awareness.

After 10 bends, resume the fundamental stance. If shaking doesn't occur after 10 minutes, do another set of bends and resume the stance. Stay with the exercise; you will have to go beyond discomfort and feelings of being tired and bored to make progress, but in time trembling and releasing will occur. Sometimes the body may even jump up and down or go into other varied moves by itself. Allow it to do so. Keep your eyes open and merely guide its direction in the space. It is very important to trust whatever the body does by itself. Just stay aware and fully experience the movements and the subsequent releases.

Hip joint release movement

First, the preliminary movement. Assume the fundamental stance. Just as you created space in the abdomen and lower rib area with the breath, take a lifting breath from the groin and get a sense of space in that area. Breathe into this area and relax the muscles in the pelvic girdle as much as you can. This will give you a warm, spacious feeling in the entire lower torso and groin. Take 10 full breaths into this area. If you do this correctly, you should feel a drop in the hip joint toward the heels, and the legs should feel longer and freer.

Now, very slowly bend forward from the hip joint (not the lumber region of the back) without shifting the weight in the feet. If your back leg muscles (hamstrings) are too tight, you may allow your knees to bend slightly. Bend down as far as you can and let your hands drop to the floor. Allow the head to dangle in toward your knees.

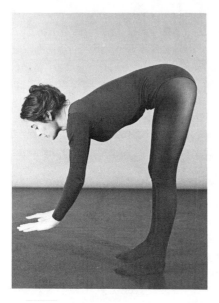 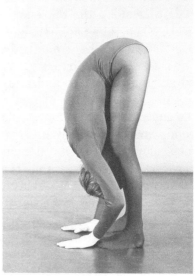

3.13, 3.14 Hip joint bend. Slowly bend forward from the hip joint, as far down as you can. Drop hands to the floor and let your head dangle in toward your knees (right).

Ideally, the bend will be so complete that the genital area, instead of stopping at the point where it is facing the floor, will actually rotate under and back and be facing behind you. You should experience a widening and opening in the upper thighs and buttocks. Stay in this position as long as you can and experience the stretching and shaking or trembling releasing action in the muscles.

Basic kick

The yogic method of kicking will not only extend the power and reach of your kick but will also help to release the leg joints and improve walking and running.

Choose a space where you have at least 12 to 15 feet to work in. Stand with your back against a wall and kick your right foot forward, turning the inside of the arch upward. Your weight

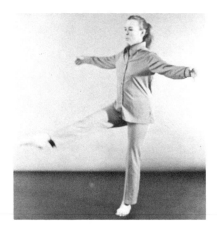
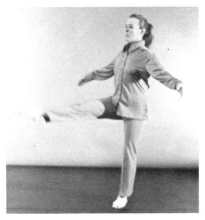

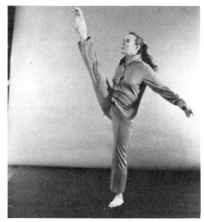

3.15, 3.16, 3.16A.   The kick. Practice low kick with weight over back leg (top, left). Now add more height to kick (top, right). Finally kick fully— notice how leg comes in toward body!

should be dropped into the ground along the outside of your left foot. As you kick, imagine the movement originating in the heel and back of the knee joint (illustration 3.15).

Be sure your leg muscles are relaxed. The standing leg muscle should not tense or move toward the kicking leg at all, and the inner thigh muscles in both legs should be relaxed throughout. Continue to kick out the right leg, varying the height of the kick from low to high. Notice that, as the kick gets higher, the legs make an arched curve that brings the thigh in toward the torso and the foot up toward the head (illustration 3.16).

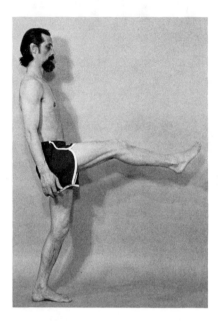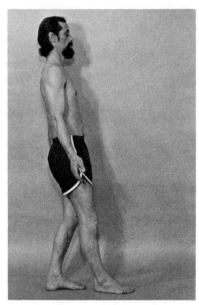

3.17, 3.18. Walking kick. Kick the right foot without shifting torso weight, buttocks, or left leg. Drop it one foot ahead of the left. Only after the right foot is in complete contact with the ground (right) should you shift your weight forward. Repeat with left leg.

If your leg muscles remain relaxed, you should experience an awareness of the true flexibility and balance in the legs. Repeat this simple exercise, kicking from high to low about 12 times with each foot. Check regularly to be sure that the standing leg is relaxed and does not move toward the kicking leg.

Walking kick

Start this exercise sitting on the edge of a hard chair with your back straight. Without leaning forward, alternately kick left foot and right foot. Return each foot to the floor before you kick out the opposite one.

Now stand and kick the right foot out without shifting the weight of the torso, buttocks or left leg forward. The sensation should be similar to the sitting kick. The torso, spine, and left leg remain stationary, with all the weight dropping into the ground along the outside of the left leg and foot. As the right foot comes down in the kick, drop it one foot ahead of the left. Only after the right foot is in complete contact with the ground should you shift your weight forward.

As you move forward on the right leg, kick the left leg out. Be sure the weight remains on the stationary leg and does not shift forward until after the kicking leg has come in full touch with the ground. As with the previous exercise, vary the height of your kick progressively from low to high. Kick in this manner for at least 10 minutes. As with all yogic movement, part of the secret to success is a full awareness of the movement coupled with yogic breathing.

Effortless walk and run

Stand in the fundamental stance and lean slightly backward into the space behind the body. Take a full storage breath, raise the ribs, and experience a slight lift in the groin area with the breath. Drop your weight into the ground through the heels, along the outsides of the feet, and extend your hands about 12 inches from the sides of your body with your palms facing forward and your fingers separated and extended.

Very slowly lift your right foot from the sole and place it down heel first, one step ahead *without taking the weight off the back leg.* Now slowly begin to shift your weight to the right foot, simultaneously moving the left foot upward and forward. Keep your attention on the sole of the foot and place it down heel first, one step ahead. Make sure the knees are relaxed. If they feel tense, allow them to bend slightly more throughout the exercise. Be sure to move from the sole and not the top of the foot, in order to help keep the ankles relaxed. Look straight ahead as you walk and experience your full peripheral vision.

As you develop a rhythm in this slow-motion walk, there should be no feeling of using the muscles deliberately to lift and move the foot upward and forward. The mere intention of moving will activate the muscles in a natural way. There should be no strain in the legs, and the foot that remains in alignment with the ground should not tense up or participate in any way as you raise the other leg. Let each leg move in its own space.

As you are moving, experience a feeling of leaning slightly backward into the space behind the body. Be aware of the back of the knee joint and get the idea of walking forward from the space behind you. Walk slowly in a large circle until you have a full, comfortable awareness of the movement; then increase the pace and complete three to four circles. Continue to increase the speed until you are walking as fast as possible without running. Allow your hands and arms to move as they please.

To increase your pace, simply speed up the rhythm of the movement; do not change it. This allows you to move faster, using the body's intelligence rather than incorporating a mental picture of rushing. If the idea of rushing dominates, there is a tendency to push forward from the neck and to lean into the

3.19, 3.20. The effortless walk. Very slowly lift right foot and place it down heel first, keeping weight on the back leg. Then slowly shift weight to the right, simultaneously moving left foot upward and forward.

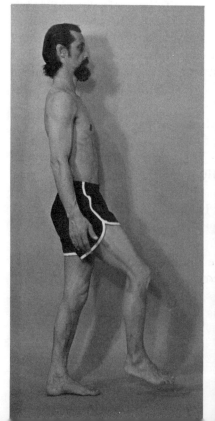
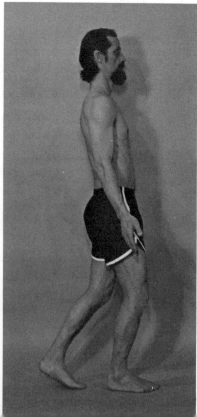

space ahead of you, pulling the weight upward and forward. Natural speed has nothing to do with rushing—it has to do with rhythm and momentum.

Once you are comfortable with a fast walking pace, shift into a run using the yogic principles. The yogic running momentum naturally carries the body along the ground from under the feet in a smooth, forward glide. Let go of any running instructions such as pumping forward with the arms. Simply allow the body to find its own natural movement.

If at any point in the exercise you notice your legs have collapsed inward or that your rib cage has fallen or your neck and head are out of alignment, slow down the movement until you regain the open, natural position you experience in the Fundamental Stance.

Jump

Whether you are jumping for height or to make a play, the perfect jump is a mixture of power and balance. A jump must take you where you want to go and return you to the ground, ready for further play. The following yogic jumping exercises will help to improve your speed, height, and balance. They also are excellent general conditioning exercises in themselves.

BASIC JUMP

Work in a space where you have at least 12 to 15 feet of floor space. Stand with the weight of your pelvis dropped into the ground through the heels, as in the basic yogic stance. Take a full storage breath. Relax your knees and squat down slightly toward the back of your heels.

Now jump straight up, springing from the outsides of the feet. Allow the weight of the legs, feet, and hips to relax toward the ground at the height of the jump, before you land on the outsides of the feet in the slightly squat position from which you started. Try to land in the exact spot from which you jumped. Take a 5-second rest between jumps.

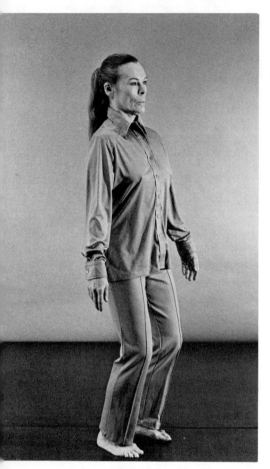 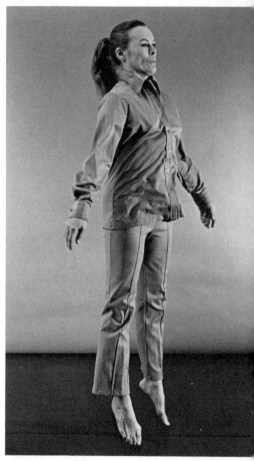

As you jump, keep your head and upper torso centered so you shoot upward directly into the space above your head. Be sure your hip girdle is relaxed and is not lifted up in back toward the lumbar region. Don't allow your chin to push up or out. Check frequently to make sure the weight is distributed along the outsides of the feet and that you have a full storage breath. The knees should be loose and relaxed. Your entire body should have a springy, loose feeling. Do about 15 stationary jumps. Then,

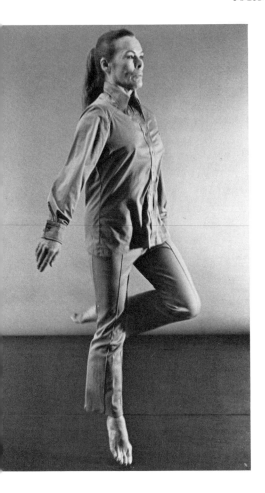

3.21, 3.21A, 3.22. The jump. Try to land on the exact spot from which you jumped.

using the same basic procedure, jump on one foot and then the other. Be sure not to lift the hip of the nonjumping leg.

MOVING JUMP

Stand facing a wall, about a foot away. Take a storage breath and prepare to do the basic jump using both feet, but instead of jumping in place, jump backward about one foot. Be sure you

start and land from a slight squat with relaxed knees, so that
the weight drops into the ground through the outsides of the legs
and feet. Execute about 20 backward jumps, and then experiment with different heights.

After you have done about 20 varied-height backward jumps,
jump forward with the sense of moving from the space behind
you.

Now play and experiment with your jumps. Place your arms
and hands in different position. Jump to the side, jumping as
high as you can and as far forward and backward as possible.
The idea is to jump and to land correctly in the slightly squat
position on the outsides of the feet, without tipping forward or
ever losing a balanced body posture.

Finally experiment by jumping forward, sideways and backward on one foot and then the other.

Advanced balancing exercises

The following exercises, the Arrow, Bow, Headstand, and
Plough, should only be attempted after you have worked and
experienced some release with the previous exercises.

Work through the following movements slowly. Don't strain
the body into the Bow and Arrow; take your time with the Head
Stand and Plough. Be sure you are doing full yogic breathing
throughout the movement.

Arrow

Bend from the hip joint. Place your palms flat on the floor and
raise your left foot all the way up and back. Now slowly "walk"
forward with the hands, as far as you can without lowering the
left leg. When you can walk no farther, lie down flat with your
hands outstretched down towards the legs.

Remain for 5 full breaths and then reverse the motion by
placing hands beside your head and walking back on your
hands, with the left foot raised. Return to the full bend position
with both hands and feet on the ground; then stand up and
repeat the exercise, raising the right foot.

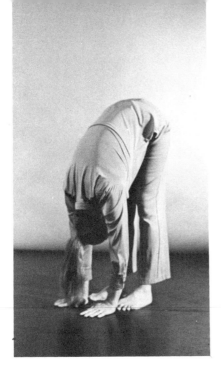

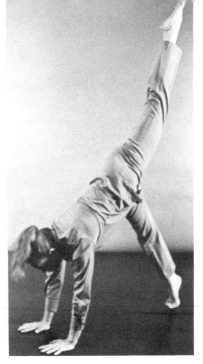

3.23A–3.23C. The arrow. The start position (left). Walk forward slowly on your hands while raising your foot as high in back as you can. Continue walking forward on your hands and bring the foot down slowly until you are lying down.

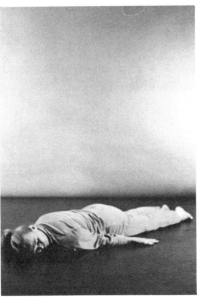

Bow

Stand on your hands and knees with your back and stomach muscles relaxed. Lift your left foot and grab it with your right hand.

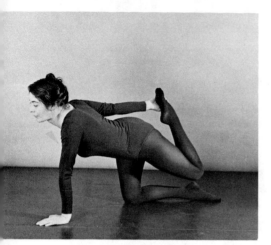 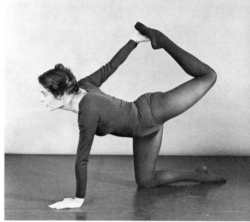

3.24, 3.25. The bow. Lift left foot and grab it with your right hand, keeping hips in a straight line with shoulders (left). Gently lift foot and stretch the back and leg muscles. Raise head and look straight ahead.

Be sure to keep your hips in a straight line with your shoulders. Without letting the torso twist to either side, gently lift the left foot and stretch the back and leg muscles. Raise your head and look straight ahead.

Hold the position for 5 full breaths and then repeat with your right leg and left hand.

HEAD STAND

Work on a soft surface, or place a small pillow on the ground for your head. Stand on your knees and elbows with your forearms flat on the ground. Interlace your fingers directly in front of your head. Now rest your head on the ground or pillow so that it is firmly clasped by your hands, as in illustration 3.26. Keep your elbows close to your ears.

"Walk" in toward the body and push up into a vertical position with the knees bent.

Try to hold the position for two minutes. If you have to use a wall for support, gently push away from the wall and try to stand free. Work several times each day until you can freely stand on your head and forearms.

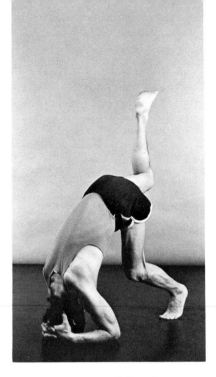

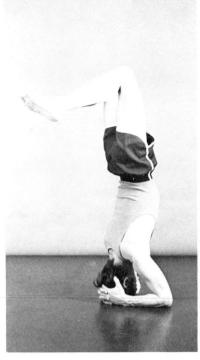

3.26. The head stand. Interlace fingers directly in front of your head and clasp head, keeping elbows close to your ears.

3.27. Use a wall if you have to.

3.28. Slowly raise heels until the legs are straight up. Balance.

3.29. Try bringing legs down with knees bent and heels meeting directly over the hands.

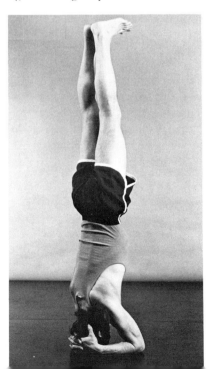

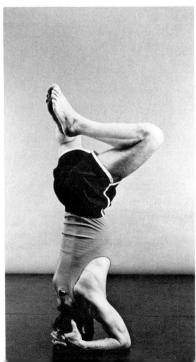

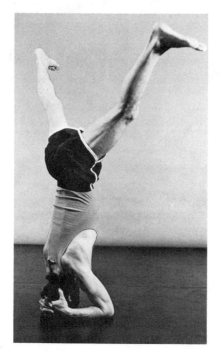

3.30. Straighten knees to form a
"Y" with the legs.

When the balance is secure, slowly raise your heels until the legs are straight up. Practice holding your balance in this position.

As your balance improves, try bringing the legs down with knees bent, thighs out to the side, and heels touching directly over the clasped hands as in illustration 3.29.

Finally, from this position straighten the knees and form a "Y" with the legs, as in illustration 3.30.

After you have mastered all four positions and can hold them comfortably, go through the entire sequence, holding each pose for about two minutes. Using your own judgment, you can experiment with longer sequences.

PLOUGH

Lie on your back and raise both feet up over the body and behind the head by supporting your hips with your hands. Keep

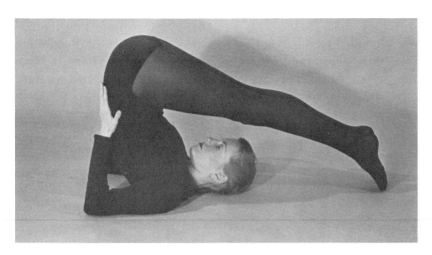

3.31. The plough. Hands supporting your hips, raise feet and keep legs parallel to the floor. Knees should be directly above the eyes as the toes touch the floor.

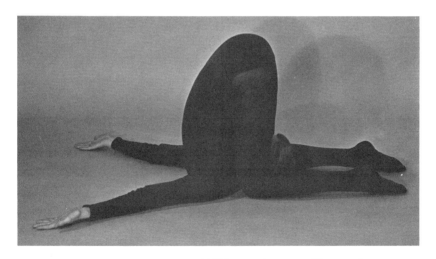

3.32. The full plough. Don't force it! With practice, you will succeed.

the legs parallel to the floor with the knees directly above your eyes. Keeping your knees straight, drop your feet directly behind your head and touch the floor with your toes, as in illustration 3.31.

If your muscles are very relaxed, you can move into the full plough (illustration 3.32) by bending the knees and bringing them to the ground directly behind the ears. Don't try to force this advanced position, but as you continue to practice, see how close you can come to performing it. One fine day, you will succeed.

4

Yogic principles for your sport

Athletes are constantly in search of optimum performance. Hence, they will adjust their style to emulate that of a more successful athlete, or to recall times when his or her own play was superior. For the most part, athletes run hot and cold in their abilities to pin down exactly what it is that makes a person play better one day than during the rest of the season.

Many believe that some athletes are "gifted," and they use this term to explain superior play. It's possible that these so-called gifted athletes have simply hit upon yoga's principles of motion and use of space without being aware of what they are doing. This is mostly unexplored territory, but we can say from experience that, as you release tension in the body and discover the yogic way of moving in the space, your performance will improve markedly.

We have organized this book in the same sequence as we present instruction to athletes at our yoga centers; we hope you will have given several hours to the basic breathing and balancing exercises before you read ahead and apply these principles to your game. *One of the more important exercises is the basic*

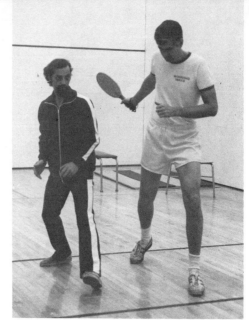

4.1. Author Harmon Hathaway, left, demonstrates proper weight distribution for racquetball or tennis to coach Garth Stam, State University College of New York.

stance combined with full yogic breathing, and we highly recommend that you spend at least 20 minutes to an hour with the stance and the breath before you start to work with your sport.

If your sport is not treated in this chapter, work with the yogic principles of related sports and apply them to your sport.

RUNNING AND JOGGING

You probably now realize that yoga is nothing more than a way of learning how to move naturally. Running is an important part in the training program of almost any sport; whether it be a long distance jog or a spirited sprint, running should be a smooth flow of motion from start to finish. In ancient China the king's messengers could run at a steady pace for days on end with little fatigue. What was their secret? The proper alignment of the body, combined with the same yogic breathing you learned earlier in this book.

In both running and jogging it is most important to have the correct relationship with the ground and with the space around the body. Most runners we have seen look as if they are falling forward when they run: The neck stretches forward; the pelvis tilts forward; the arms violently punch into the space ahead of

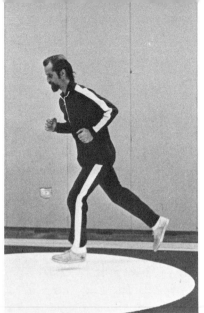 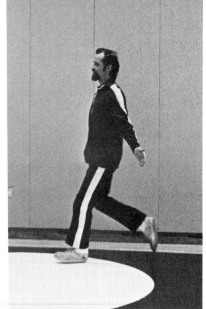

4.2. The strained running or jogging position.

4.3. The yogic running or jogging position. Note the differences.

the body. Such strain wastes valuable energy and throws the runner off balance.

Notice in illustrations 4.2 and 4.3 the difference between the natural yogic running position and the strained position of many runners, both amateurs and professionals. The forward strain often results from the runner's attitude: He wants to be better and faster, and he struggles to reach the finish line or struggles to keep in shape. This is another example of how the mind, grasping an idea like success, can actually interfere with the natural, efficient movement of the body.

In the yogic position, notice the natural tilt of the pelvis, the relaxed position of the arms, and the easy way the head and neck sit on the shoulders in proper alignment with the spine. This posture is similar to the basic yogic stance described in the preceding chapter. In yogic running, the upper body actually feels like a rider sitting in the saddle of the pelvis. The legs do all the action; there should be no effort to pump ahead with the arms. In fact, the arms should hang loosely until they find their own rhythm in response to the action of the legs.

If you have done a lot of jogging and running without practicing yoga, there is a good chance your body moves in the strained position. If this is so, bad running habits are maintained by tension in your muscles. The exercises in this chapter will free the muscles so you can comfortably assume the yogic running position. This natural position will give you greater endurance, speed, and power. Try to find locations where you may jog or run on soft ground.

FREEING THE KNEES

Lie on your back, with two or three firm pillows under your buttocks so your pelvis is angled upward. Tuck in your chin so that it touches your chest; extend your arms to the sides, palms up. Now lift your right foot off the ground until the right leg is perpendicular to the ground. As you lift, be sure the stomach muscles are used as little as possible. Now lift the left foot until both legs are perpendicular to the ground. Without altering the position of the thighs or pelvis, slowly lower the feet, bringing the heels all the way down to the buttocks.

Concentrate on the movement of the feet and imagine them to be the source of motion. Now slowly raise the feet, extending them again to the upright position without altering the position of the pelvis. Repeat this simple up-and-down motion and be sure you are doing full yogic breathing.

Sooner or later you will feel a shaking in the legs, through the pelvis, and along the spine. The shaking is the actual loosening of the running muscles. The more intense the shaking, the greater the release of pent-up energies. We have found, when doing this exercise, that there is usually one area of movement where the shaking is greatest. When you find this area, confine the up-and-down motion to it and allow the shaking to travel throughout your body.

This simple exercise is amazingly effective, especially when it is practiced for long periods of time. You should do this exercise for at *least 20 minutes* and preferably longer. You may also do this exercise without pillows.

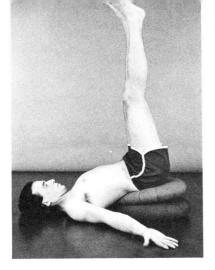

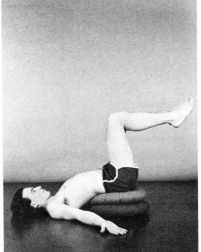

4.4–4.6. Freeing the knees. Lift legs one at a time, using stomach muscles as little as possible. Slowly lower legs, bringing heels all the way down to the buttocks. Use yogic breathing.

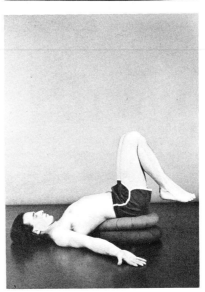

FREEING THE HIPS AND THIGHS

Here's an equally effective variation on the previous exercise that reaches into different muscle groups. Again, try to practice for at least 20 minutes. Lie on your back, with a firm pillow or two under your buttocks so that your pelvis is angled upward. Tuck in your chin so that it touches your collarbone, and extend your arms comfortably out from the sides of your body. Now lift

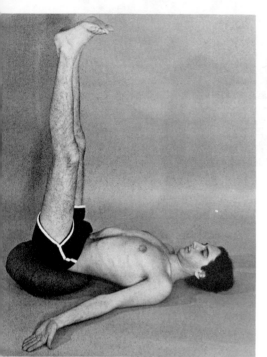
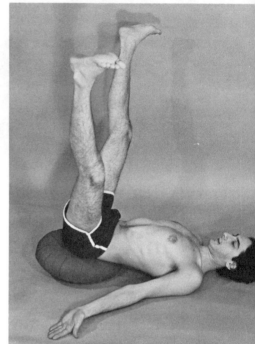

4.7–4.9.   Freeing the hips and thighs. A variation on the preceding exercise, this one moves up the body.

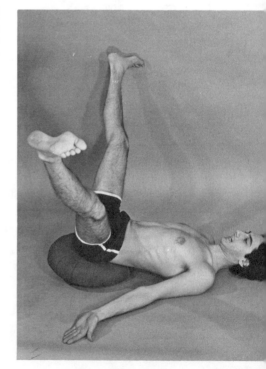

your right foot off the ground until the right leg is perpendicular to the ground. Then lift the left foot until both legs are perpendicular to the ground. The ankle joint should be directly above the hip joint, and the legs should be straight. If you find it difficult to straighten the knee, place more pillows under the pelvis so you can get the legs as straight as possible. Now turn the feet at the ankle so your soles are angled toward one another. Slowly move the feet apart to get as large a "V" shape as possible without straining the groin muscles. Then bring the feet slowly back together until they touch.

ALIGNING THE BODY

Stand in the basic yogic position, with the weight radiating down the lateral edge of the body and into the ground, mostly through the heels. Now raise your right foot; notice the sensation in the foot as it comes off the ground. As soon as the foot is

4.10, 4.11. Aligning the body. Lift from the foot, not the leg, in order to retrain your legs how to walk.

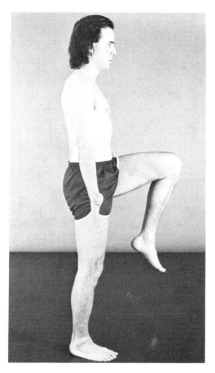
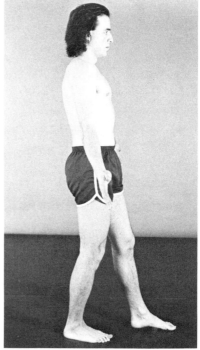

raised, the ankle should feel loose. Lift the left foot high, bringing the knee up toward the chest as in illustrations 4.10 and 4.11. Now slowly lower the foot and place it on the ground one step ahead of the right foot.

As soon as the left foot touches the ground, raise the right foot and repeat the motion. Continue to "walk" in this manner. With each step, be aware that each leg moves independently of the other. Feel the entire weight of the body along the outside of the stationary leg and foot. Be sure the stationary leg makes no effort to help raise the other leg.

As with the previous exercise, you will eventually notice a shaking in the thighs and lower back. Try to increase the shaking by doing the exercise more slowly. Practice for at least 20 minutes.

4.12. Running in slow motion. Throw the foot out, as if you were kicking off a shoe.

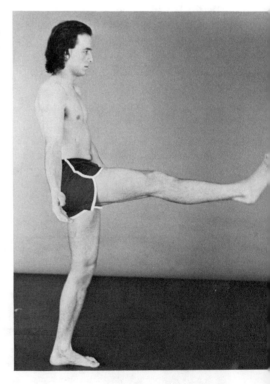

RUNNING IN SLOW MOTION

Stand in the basic yogic position and lift your right foot about 12 inches off the ground. Then throw the foot out, as if you were kicking off a shoe (illustration 4.12).

Now return the right foot to the ground, one step ahead of the left, and repeat the raising and kicking motion with the left foot. Practice this exercise slowly for at least 20 minutes; gradually increase your speed until you are jogging and then running. Stop running the minute you notice you are in a strained position, and start the exercise all over again.

If possible, find an hour each day and go through these three exercises, either in your free time or, better yet, just before you run. If you do these exercises faithfully, you will soon be running in the yogic position and reaping the benefits: greater endurance, speed, and enjoyment.

SWIMMING

Swimming is one of the best all-around exercises, for it utilizes every muscle without putting an undue stress on any

4.13. Harmon Hathway, right, works poolside with Olympic swimming coach Lee Abbot.

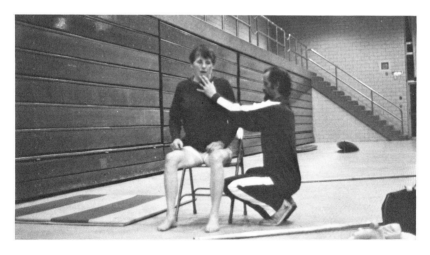

part of the body. Competition swimming, however, demands an exceptionally high level of fitness and endurance; it can lead to psycho-muscular tensions when the body is not properly aligned. The swimmer will find that full yogic breathing will develop his or her endurance and increase buoyancy. The basic yogic exercises for balance will improve alignment in the water.

You should have practiced full yogic breathing for at least 10 hours before you attempt to adapt it to the water. As the rhythm of yogic breathing becomes natural, you will discover that your body will adjust it to your stroke and speed. Remember, you can practice yogic breathing anytime: walking, sitting, lying down, or standing.

RACING START AND TURN

As you prepare for your racing dive, bend from the hip and upper leg joint with as little roundness in the spine as possible. This will place most of the upper body weight in front of the legs and will give a more consistent and a straighter line to your dive.

As the body moves forward in the dive, push off from the outside of the feet. Evenness and balance are important, because they give the body two equal lines of pressure for the spring and

4.14. The racing dive. Bend from the hip, not the waist, for a more consistent, straighter-line dive.

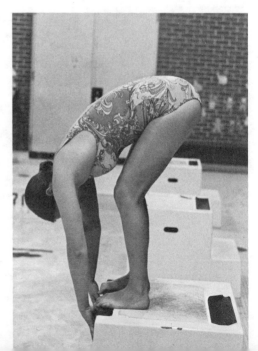

help to prevent a roll in the dive. If the feet are not pointing straight forward, there is a tendency to push from the inside of the foot; this creates a narrower line of balance through the center of the body and increases the possibility of a roll.

TURN

Although there are different turns for different strokes, we will discuss the turn in general, because the yogic principles involved are the same for each type.

When you plant your feet in your normal turn, make sure the outsides of the feet touch the wall equally. This will prevent any slipping and will ensure an even push so that the body moves in a straight line from the wall. In most cases, swimmers do not distinguish which part of the foot hits the wall; in many cases the preference is to use the large ball of the foot (illustrations 4.15 and 4.16).

The push, of course, comes from the whole foot, but your attention should be on the *outsides* of the feet. As you move away

4.15, 4.16. The turn. Using the toes, or the balls of the feet (top), doesn't give you the power that the feet flat against the wall will give you.

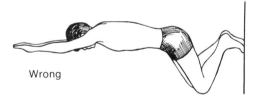

Wrong

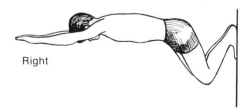

Right

from the wall, the legs should not be locked but should instead be stretched back without effort. In the push off, the knees should not touch or be pulled toward each other, since this would limit the straight-ahead power of the push. Experiment with the distance between your feet as you push off to discover the position where you get your maximum thrust.

JUMP

This exercise, done out of the water, will help you to get in touch with the correct use of the muscles that are important to your turn.

Begin by standing in the basic stance, with your weight

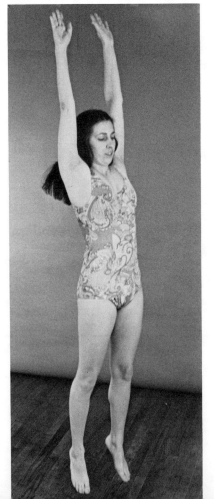

4.17.   The jump. Perfect this on the ground, and you will increase the power of your turns in the water.

toward the outsides of the feet and heels and your buttocks relaxed. Breathe comfortably. Your arms should be relaxed and your palms open. Now, bend the knees slightly, so your heels remain on the ground, and then push lightly against the ground with the outsides of the feet; straighten the leg without the knees' locking. Notice that by simply increasing the pressure against the ground, the leg straightens without effort. Repeat this bending and straightening motion and permit any shaking or trembling that might occur in the legs. Finally, to get a sense of balanced power, jump straight up from the slightly bent position and shoot your arms over head to help with the lift.

Ideally, you will land exactly where you left the floor. When the body is up in the air, let the ankles relax, toes pointed downward. There should be no discernible tension in the body when you are up in the air. The feet should be about 8 to 10 inches apart, and as you are ascending, the legs should move together naturally. Repeat this until you get a sense of relaxation while you jump and the confidence that you can transfer this relaxation to your swimming turn.

Breathing in the Water

This exercise will be done in the water as you float on your back.

Take a full storage breath and start panting at a comfortable rate. Remember: This is *not* a recommended swimming breath. It is an exercise breath to increase the lung capacity. While you are floating, let the body relax completely, with your legs

4.18. Yogic breathing in the water. Full storage breath with panting increases your swimming breaths.

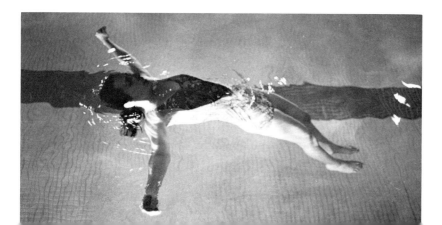

hanging down, arms relaxed, and palms open as in illustration 4.18.

STROKE

You can't benefit fully from the following exercise unless you already have a thorough mastery of your stroke—and have done several hours of yogic breathing and standing. The idea here is to try to experience the full, open sensation of the yogic stance and to transfer that sensation to your movement in water.

When you are swimming, try to feel the external lines of the body from the toes up through the outside fingers. When you

4.19. The yogic stance. Lift the body by pressing from the outsides of your hands. Use this same outside line of force for a more powerful swimming stroke.

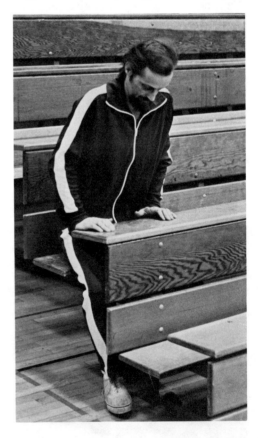

catch and recover, you should use the muscles that come into play when you pull and push from this outside line. This is the same principle that is illustrated by sitting at a table or a bench and pushing down against it with the outside of the hand so you lift your body off the chair, as in illustration 4.19.

Now try the same movement by pressing with the *inside* of the hand and arm. You will notice the difference in strength that the outside push has over the inside push. Apply this principle in the water by being aware of the outside lines of the body.

This same yogic principle holds true for the kick. As you work out, be aware of using the outside of the legs. This will give you greater balance in the water and will keep the body straighter.

To maintain flexibility in the muscles, swimmers should experiment with all of the releasing exercises in chapter 5.

DIVING

Diving requires a remarkable combination of muscular control, relaxation, and balance. Full yogic breathing will give your body a lighter, springier feeling; the yogic stance will help develop the fine sense of balance essential to the diver. Here the basics are not only important, they also are essential. The diver should practice breathing and standing daily as part of his regular training program.

APPROACH

When you practice the approach on dry land, you should begin by standing in the basic yogic stance with weight on the outsides of the feet. This will keep the body in a straight line through the hurdle and entrance into the dive.

This exercise will help you get a sense of relaxation in the legs and calf. You can then transfer this sense to your approach.

Stand as if you were starting an approach and press into the ground with the outsides of the feet, allowing the heels to rise slowly until you are standing on the outside balls of the feet (illustration 4.20).

Maintain a relaxed leg and calf throughout the movement. First try this holding onto some object, until you can stand on the ball of the foot with a completely relaxed—not limp—leg. Then practice the exercise in place or while walking around. If necessary, allow your legs to wiggle or shake in order to facilitate relaxation in the calf and upper leg muscles. Do this for about 5 minutes each time.

HURDLE

The leading leg in the hurdle must move freely in its own space, without tension but with enough force so that it adds to your height. Many athletes have the musculature of their legs somewhat tied together, so that when one leg rises the other moves with it. This threatens balance and needs to be corrected. (Basic yogic breathing will expand the internal space in the

4.20. The approach. Keep the legs and calf muscles relaxed.

4.21. The hurdle. Keep the body straight as the knee comes up, and breathe deeply.

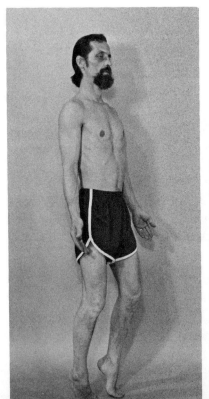

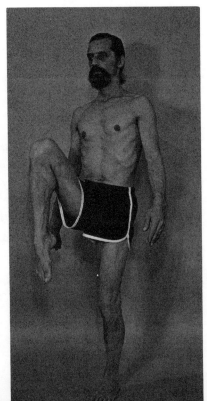

abdomen and create greater flexibility and independence for the hips and legs.)

Stand in the basic stance and breathe deeply; raise one foot at a time, bringing the knee up toward the chest. Keep your awareness on maintaining a relaxed standing leg. When you can raise your legs independently of one another, begin to work on your hurdle.

Start from the basic stance and practice the hurdle on a trampoline or on the board. Be sure the full weight of the body falls into the ground through the outside edge of the standing foot. The full potential of the hurdle can also be inhibited by the upper body pressing forward against the lead leg. As you practice, be sure that your spine is straight and that you are bringing the leg in toward the body and not kicking it out.

TAKING OFF

At this point in the dive, and until you reach the peak, you still want to maintain a straight, balanced line to the body.

If possible, work on a trampoline. Stand for a few minutes in the basic stance and then jump up and down; try to maintain the open, spacious feeling of the stance as you move. Keep the legs relaxed under the body as you are in the air. When the body line is straight, there will be no need to tense the legs together.

DIVE

The first position we will examine is the *pike*. You may already do this correctly, or you may hit the pike perfectly sometimes and not other times. The idea here is to add consistency to the dive by being relaxed and by discovering the most balanced position for your body.

Stand in the basic yogic position with your knees slightly flexed and bend forward from the upper leg joint rather than from the waist (See illustration 4.22). Experiment. Bend correctly from the leg joint, then incorrectly from the waist, so you can feel the subtle difference. After you have understood the

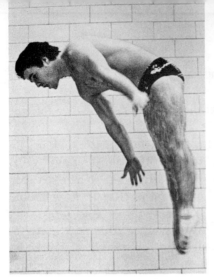 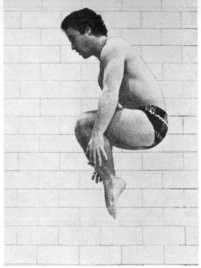

4.22. Pike position. Bend from the hip joint not from the waist. Jack Walsh, five-time NCAA finalist.

4.23. The tuck. Jack Walsh.

correct bend, work on the trampoline to perfect this movement in action.

The tuck position can also be refined by working on the trampoline. Make sure your body remains straight as you bring your legs up to the tuck position. The knees should move up and in toward the body, as in illustration 4.23.

As you initiate the lift in the tuck position, you should feel as if you are moving the heel and foot toward the buttocks. By simply placing your attention on raising the heel and foot, you will rid yourself of trying to lift the leg and thus creating tension where none is needed. When coming out of the tuck, you should experience the same relaxed feeling of just moving the feet through space.

TENNIS

Tennis, like bowling or golf, is a game that gives millions of people the opportunity to engage in healthy exercise and social enjoyment. The popularity of tennis continues to grow in America, involving more people every year. Yet, of all the people playing, perhaps only 5 percent could be called professional or even highly skilled. Both the professional and the amateur can benefit by applying yogic principles to their game. In some cases, professionals are already using these principles, but many are probably unaware of what they are doing.

We will not be addressing racket work per se and advise amateurs to read up on this skill or to work with a tennis pro. Our main emphasis is in developing *optimum balance, power,* and *relaxation* through yogic movement in order to improve both game and body.

To begin, we advise that everyone do basic yogic breathing as described in chapter 1. The professional, especially, should practice for many hours, since this breathing will be a real benefit to his or her game. When a full understanding of yogic breathing becomes natural, your endurance, awareness, timing, and recovery will improve.

You can work basic yogic breathing into your training by practicing the exercise below. (You should have first worked at least 5 hours on the breathing exercises described in chapter 1.)

BREATHING WHILE PLAYING

This exercise can be done with a partner across court or alone by volleying against a wall.

Take a full storage breath before play begins and continue to do full yogic breathing throughout the volley. Concentrate on the breath and keep the play simple to start. Work this way for about 15 minutes. If you lose the storage breath, or if it feels as if it wants to let go, stop play for a few minutes while you practice breathing; then resume your volley. As you play, allow the breath to stretch from the lower abdomen area all the way up through the chest and around the back. Proper breathing will help you keep your back straight and therefore less tense.

MOVING WITH EASE

This next exercise will show how to move from side to side and forward and backward in the most efficient, energy-conserving fashion. To the professional, balance and speed are very important; moving while applying yogic principles will give you both, even as you expend less energy.

Stand in the ready position, with the weight of the body on the outsides of the feet and slightly back toward the heels. This will keep the body in full touch with the ground, rather than waiting on the balls of the feet which creates unnecessary tension before moving. (See illustrations 4.24 and 4.25.)

Your knees should be flexed in preparation for action but with minimal upper leg tension. The upper body should be straight, with the breath full. You can adjust the upper body's position to suit your own preferences during matches. However, in this exercise, work with the upper body straight over the legs and feet. Now thrust the right leg to the side with a feeling of just moving the foot out, as in illustration 4.26.

4.24, 4.25. Waiting with ease. In the ready position, the body should be erect and balanced (left), not leaning forward and tense.

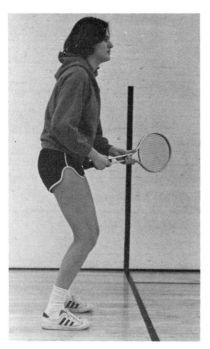 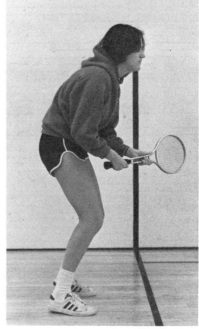

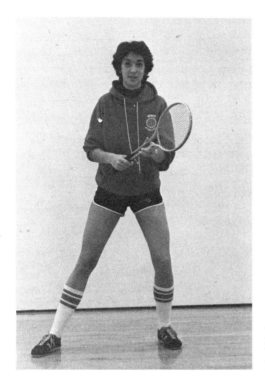

4.26. Moving with ease. The right leg slides out, with the body weight remaining on the left.

Get the idea of moving from the sole of the foot—not the top of the foot. This is a very important point: The foot leads, and if you put your attention on the foot instead of on the leg there is automatically less effort in moving the body. When you put the right foot out, start your push from the outside of the left foot. The left foot then follows by sliding rapidly toward the right foot. Move very slowly to one side, so that you are aware of putting the lead foot out and pushing from the outside of the trailing leg. You should also be aware of the trailing foot's movement as it comes into place for the next step.

As you practice and become more familiar with the ease with which the feet move, you can increase the pace from side to side. After you have worked sideways and are well acquainted with the foot action, start to work in the same manner while you move around the court in all directions.

POWER AND BALANCE

To develop power in your tennis play, you must learn to use the action of the soles of the feet against the ground.

Work with a racket. Stand in place and make the forehand stroke, pushing against the ground with the outside of the back foot. As you move forward, the weight of the body transfers to the outside of the front foot. Move in this way, with the weight on the outsides of the feet for both the backhand and forehand strokes. (See illustrations 4.27 and 4.28.)

With a little practice, the distribution of weight along the outsides of the feet will come to feel natural; when used in your game, this new balance will increase power and balance.

GOLF

The golfer spends only a fraction of his time actually hitting the ball; most of his time is spent walking from one shot to another. Walking time provides an invaluable opportunity to relax and to

4.27, 4.28. Power and balance. For both the forehand (left) and the backhand, notice that the weight remains in the back leg before the swing.

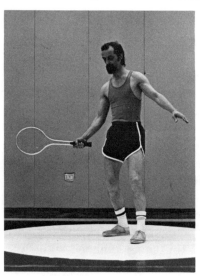
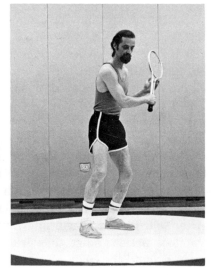

prepare the body for the next shot. Once you learn to apply basic principles of yoga, you should be able to arrive at the 18th hole without the fatigue that results from many hours of poor posture.

Every golfer should review and master the yogic principles outlined in chapters 1 and 3. This understanding will lay the groundwork for refining your golfing technique. The section on jogging and running will be useful in training and for unlearning poor physical habits.

Loosening up

Whenever you work out, you should be doing yogic walking and breathing. Stand for a few minutes in the basic yogic posture and do some deep breathing until you feel a correct alignment in the body. Now, slowly take a step forward and be sure your foot lands on the outside of the heel first and then on the outside of the foot. Your knees should be slightly bent, and your feet should point straight forward. Be sure to maintain your storage breath and full yogic breathing. Continue to walk slowly, and gradually increase your speed to a normal pace.

Once a walking and breathing rhythm has been established, the rate of breathing may change. So may the style of your walk: Let this occur. Permit the body to trot, march, or run as it wishes. The idea is to allow the body itself to loosen up and shake off tension—and habit.

The golf swing

One of the most important elements to a successful golf swing is bringing the knees and hips around *before* you hit the ball, in order to get full power. Most pros teach this with varying success, but in many cases there is an awkward turning of the body or a choppy motion that persists. Either results in inconsistent swings.

This exercise will help take the inconsistency out of your swing. It can be done anywhere there is enough room to swing your arms freely. Take the usual stance for the driving swing, with your weight distributed equally through both feet. Holding an imaginary golf club, draw your arms back and shift the weight onto the *outside* of the back foot so that all your weight is distributed along the outer edge of the foot.

As you reach the top of your swing, shift your weight onto the outside edge of the front foot. The knees and hips will follow naturally as a result of this shift, but your concentration should remain on your feet—not on your knees and hips. Repeat the swing a number of times, each time initiating the motion with a shift of the weight from the outside of one foot to the outside of the other.

Many teachers say that you should position the weight on the inside of the back foot to increase "torque." Not only is this inconsistent with the general principles of yoga, but it also limits the amount of arc the swing generates and can lead to tension in the ankle, knee, and hip of the back leg. However, for a golfer to make such a change may be very difficult; he or she should experiment with our position to see if it adds to the distance and consistency of the golf shots. Our primary interest here is to get you used to feeling the ground with the feet and transferring the

4.28–4.30. The golf swing. The weight moves to the outside edge of the back foot as the arms begin the swing. The hips will follow.

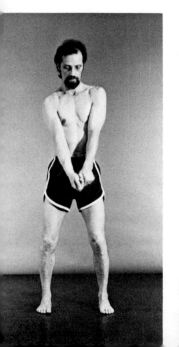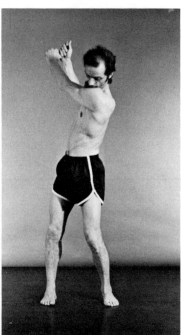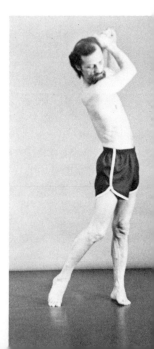

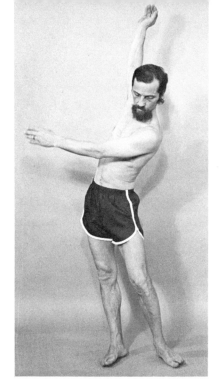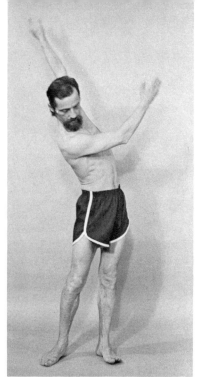

4.31, 4.32. Golf Relaxer. Shift the weight from the outside of one foot to the outside of the other; let the arms and body sway as if you were swinging a club.

weight of the body from the back of the body to the front of the body without moving in segments. This will occur if you feel the ground throughout the exercise. Once the yogic swing position is mastered, you should notice both greater accuracy and distance in your drives. The same principles should be used at all times, even when you have to hit out of a bunker.

GOLF RELAXER

The following exercise is designed to loosen you up and to work out tensions that may interfere with your golf swing.

Stand with feet apart in the basic driving stance, but with your hands apart. Now shift the weight from the outside of one foot to the outside of the other and back again, in a rocking motion. Let the arms and body sway as if you were swinging a club in both directions so that the momentum to the left and right are equally balanced. As you are swaying, use deep yogic

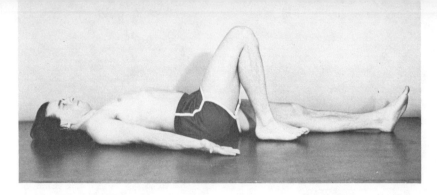

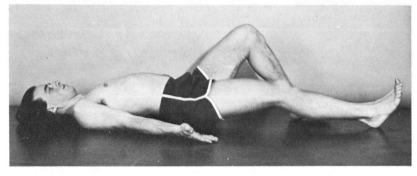

4.33, 4.34. Before and after skiing. Slide the heel up, allow the leg to shoot out and drop, and repeat with other leg.

breathing and feel a stretch in the torso and shoulders. Allow the arms to swing as fully as possible; don't prevent the movement from changing or from becoming excessive. Trust the body. The purpose of this exercise is to stretch and relax the muscles used when swinging. Experiment with this relaxing swing for 5 minutes or longer.

SKIING

Skiing can provide people of all ages with the healthful, enjoyable pleasure of moving along nature's grand white robe— or it can strain muscles and break bones. The secret to good and safe skiing is balance and control. For this reason, all of the exercises in chapter 3 should be practiced repeatedly by the skier. The aim is to transfer the open, balanced sensation of the fundamental stance to your skiing posture. This can happen of its own accord once you are comfortable with the yogic approach to standing, walking, and running described in chapter 3.

BEFORE AND AFTER

In comfortable clothing, lie down on a mat or rug and do a minute or two of full breathing. Then slide the heel of one leg up toward the buttocks (illustrations 4.33 and 4.34).

Now allow the leg to shoot out easily and flop toward the floor in a straight line. While the near leg is dropping, the other heel starts up toward the buttocks in preparation for dropping. The legs are alternately moved and dropped to the floor with a resounding thump. This will loosen the stiff inner muscles of the leg, increase the circulation in the legs, and ready them for skiing—or relax them after skiing.

FREEING THE LEGS

Lie on your back and raise both feet up over the body and behind the head by supporting your hips with your hands. Keep the legs parallel to the floor with the knees directly above your eyes, as in illustration 4.35.

Hol⁻¹ the position for 20 minutes and allow any shaking and releasing action to occur.

THE KNEE DROP

Sink into the basic yoga knee bend, as described in the Fundamental Stance, with your arms extended. Bring the buttocks down toward the heels and hold the position for a second.

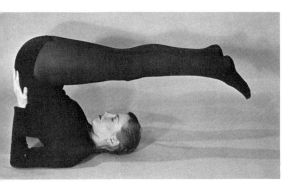

4.35. Freeing the legs. Hold this position and allow the shaking and releasing action to occur.

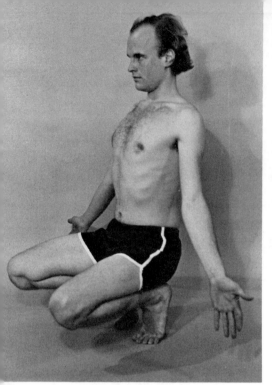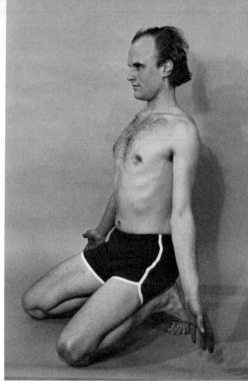

4.36, 4.37. The knee drop. This exercise increases flexibility in the feet, legs, and buttocks. From the knee bend, roll forward and then backward.

Now roll forward from the bottom of your feet and gently land on your knees. Then roll back, using the outside balls of the feet. Do 10 to 20 knee drops. (If you experience a stretching pain in the balls of the feet, use your own judgment as to how many drops to perform. Yoga should not be painful.) As you continue to practice this exercise, you will experience additional flexibility in the feet, legs, and buttocks.

BOWLING

More than 60 million Americans bowl. Yet, there is very little guidance for either the professional or the amateur. Every bowler knows the pleasure of getting a strike; perhaps some can even feel a strike in the body before the ball hits the pins. But few know how to roll strike after strike. To a yoga master this is surprising, since there is only one variable in bowling—the way you throw the ball. There is no opponent working against you;

there are no surprises, no curves, no variables in wind or weather. As in archery, if the shot can be perfected, the arrow should hit the bull's-eye every time. We honestly believe that if you work regularly with the fundamental breathing and balancing exercises in the first three chapters and then apply them to your game as we suggest below, you can expect remarkable results—maybe even a perfect game.

APPROACH

Probably the biggest mistake a bowler makes is trying to *throw* the ball, rather than allowing the momentum of the ball to do the work. The approach and the release of the ball should be one smooth motion. The walk should be in a perfectly straight and balanced line, with no wobble or deviation.

At first, work without a ball. Start from the basic yogic stance, step forward in your approach, with the weight of the body remaining on the back leg. As in the yogic walk, don't shift your weight forward until the lead foot has touched the ground. Keep the feet pointed straight ahead, the breath full, and the spine straight.

Slowly practice your approach and be aware of the weight on the outsides of the feet. Gradually increase the speed of your

4.38–4.40. The approach. Weight is aligned on the outsides of the feet. The swing is steady, and the hand and ball, rather than the arm, lead.

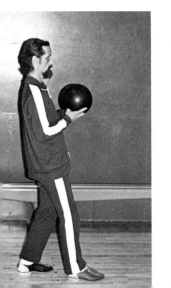 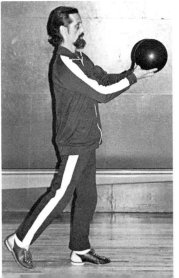 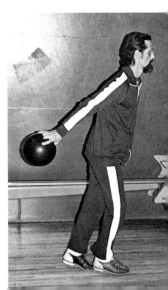

walk until you find a comfortable rhythm. Once you feel you are breathing fully and your walk is aligned and balanced, begin working with a ball.

Keep the ball centered in front of the body as you walk forward. After you put the ball forward allow it to swing back freely. As the ball comes forward, be aware of keeping the weight on the outside of the lead foot. You should feel as though the hand and ball are coming forward, rather than the arm. This awareness will prevent the upper arm from tensing. In this way, too, you will gradually find the natural rhythm you need without throwing the ball or becoming tense.

FINAL STEP

This is where most bowlers go wrong. Ideally, you should actually slide forward on this step; in any event, you must keep your feet pointed straight forward and the body balanced on the lead foot. Don't allow the action of the ball to pull you off balance. If it does, you are trying to throw the ball.

4.41, 4.42.   The final step. The spine is straight, and the torso doesn't twist to the side. Bend the forward knee, and continue to use yogic breathing.

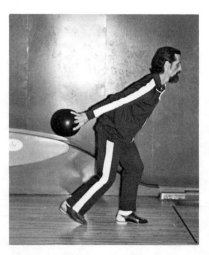 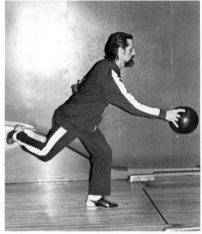

To improve this important step, stand with your finishing foot forward and let the ball swing back and forth at your side. Balance on the forward foot and let the back foot move as if you were actually letting the ball go. Keep the spine straight and don't allow the torso to twist to the side as the ball comes forward. Let the knee of the forward foot bend and the body dip each time the ball swings forward. The idea here is to become used to proper balance and breathing while swinging the ball. Stay with the exercise until this occurs naturally.

If you continue to apply basic yogic breathing and balance to your game, you will increase the consistency of your play and finish the game feeling invigorated.

FOOTBALL

The football player is subject to numerous physical problems arising from the aggressive nature of the game. Injuries and tensions can result due to constant body impact. Brute power is certainly important in many instances; yet, we all know that great play requires a flexible, agile body on the field. The ability to dance through the space, whether it be in blocking or handling the ball, brings about the spectacular plays that distinguish the great player from the ordinary. This is where yoga can make its greatest contribution to your game.

If you have already begun to practice the basic breathing and balancing exercises in the first three chapters of this book, you are on your way to a more nimble and less injury-prone game. Yogic breathing should be used at all times. Obviously, when you are in the middle of play, your attention should be on the game, but during a huddle or waiting for the line of scrimmage to form, be aware of your breathing and consciously use the breath to relax and energize the body. Since most play takes only several seconds and the periods between plays last considerably longer, there are numerous opportunities during a game to bring about relaxation and recovery. Next time on the field, make a point of using your free time to relax, align, and vitalize the body by applying the breathing and balancing principles of

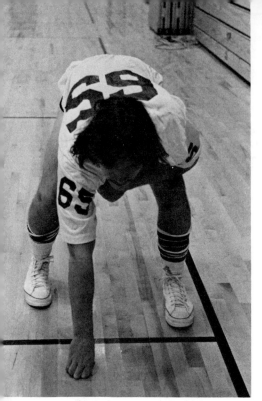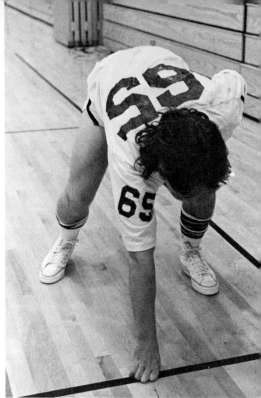

4.43, 4.44. Line play. The feet should be straight ahead (left), with the weight evenly balanced. When weight is on the inside of the back foot (right), power is decreased.

yoga. If you practice consistently, you will find you are far less tired at the end of a game.

Exercise for Line Play

This exercise can be done alone pushing against a solid object, with a practice sled, or with a teammate. Begin without equipment, working slowly until you have understood the fine points of the exercise.

Stand in the three-point stance and simply practice deep yogic breathing for a few minutes. Feel the breath reaching down to the lower ribs, abdomen, and hips. Point your feet straight ahead, with the weight of the body going into the ground through the outsides of the feet, as in illustrations 4.43 and 4.44. Keep the body relaxed so there is an even feeling between all three points on the ground. Then give yourself the command to move, and start pushing against the ground from the outsides of the feet. As you step forward or backward, make sure the outside of the raised foot hits the ground hard as it comes down. You should feel the push from the ground, going into the object you are pushing against and along the outside of the body. This is different from feeling a single line of force through the center of the body. This new sensation will widen the blocking area and maintain your power from shoulder to shoulder. When you watch football on the field or on television, notice that some linemen push from inside the balls of the feet—and that theirs are often the blocks that fail.

To distinguish the difference, try to block both ways, first with the weight on the insides and then on the outsides of the feet. The difference in your power may surprise you.

The principles of yoga described for line play also apply to the running backs. The important factor is the distribution of the weight along the outsides of the feet.

Exercise for running

The ideas behind this exercise are efficient use of the ground for power and elimination of unnecessary muscular effort.

Stand directly in front of a hard chair (or stairs), with the

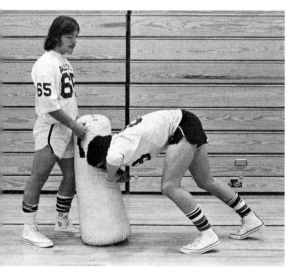

4.45.   Line play. Push and power come from the ground and legs, not from the upper body.

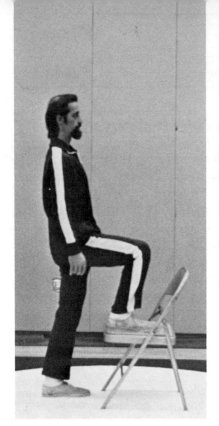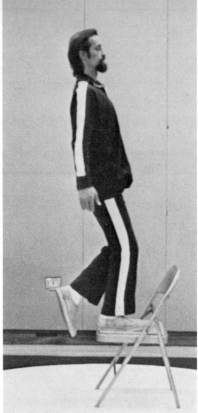

4.46, 4.47. Exercise for running. The body maintains its straight, balanced line—and the runner learns to climb or to run up stairs without wasted effort.

weight relaxed into the ground along the outsides of the feet and with your knees slightly bent. Now lift the right foot high and come down hard on the chair with the sole of that foot; continue to put pressure into the chair as your body rises up. Stand straight over the left foot until you rise up onto the chair and the left foot naturally swings up to join the right foot on the chair, as in illustrations 4.46 and 4.47.

The idea is to develop a smooth, single motion without leaning forward, so that the body naturally swings up into a standing position. Step straight down with the left foot, without tensing the leg muscles, and land with the weight on the outside of the foot. Bring the right leg down and repeat the exercise, rising on the left leg. Once you have perfected a single, smooth motion, you can climb or run up stairs by trying to maintain the same sensation of pushing *against* the stairs. After awhile, you should be able to ascend rapidly without wasted effort.

In addition to the above exercise, all players should practice the exercises in the running and jogging section of this chapter.

BACKWARD SLIDING RUN

This exercise is not only useful in football, particularly for the defensive backs, but also for developing coordination and balance in all sports. If possible, practice around a track; use light gear and wear sneakers to start. Later you may want to work out with heavier gear and shoes.

Assume the basic stance described in chapter 3 and lean backward, as if you are falling. Now "catch" the body by placing one foot after the other on the ground behind the body. This action will occur naturally. The moving foot should only lift slightly off the ground and should first touch on the outside of the heel. Let the feet slide, rather than actually step, back. This backward sliding action will leave the toes, the front part of the feet, and the legs more relaxed than the pumping action com-

4.48, 4.49. Backward run. Lean back (left) and then "catch" the body. This can make stopping and changing direction much easier on the football field.

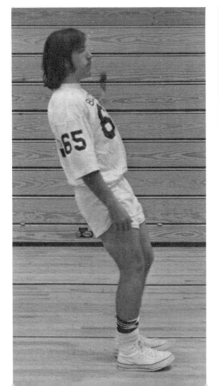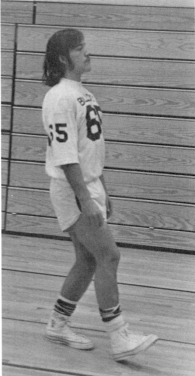

mon to many runners. The knees should be bent slightly and the
arms should hang loosely at the sides. The breathing should be
full but not strained. Begin this exercise slowly in order to
become comfortable with the sliding motion and footing. When
the movement feels natural, increase your speed by leaning
farther backward. As you move faster and faster, you may reach
a point where the body feels as if it is going out of control.
Should this happen, slow down, and then slowly increase your
speed again. In time you will be able to raise your speed control
threshold.

Once you are comfortable moving backward in this way,
introduce other moves that a defensive back must master, such
as stopping suddenly and moving laterally. The backward sliding run makes stopping and changing direction much easier
than the backward pumping run.

RELAXING THE BACK MUSCLES

One of the reasons football players have back problems is that
they tend to block with the upper body instead of using the
whole body, from the ground up. The sensation of a balanced
body gained from yogic walking, standing, and running will
help to eliminate this tendency. The following exercise is designed to release accumulated tension in the back through
trembling and shaking rather than through harsh stretching.

Stand in the basic yogic stance with your knees relaxed, and
bend forward from the hips, not the waist. Let your head hang
and allow the neck muscles to relax. Now take a full breath and
feel the action of the inhale expand all the way along the spine.
Breathe deeply in this position for at least 10 minutes, and allow
the breath to expand the lower back ribs. If the body starts to
bob up and down or sway from side to side, go with the motion.
Try to experience the body with the breath from the inside out,
and stretch the entire torso with this breath.

If you practice long enough, you will experience a trembling
along the spine and down into the buttocks and legs. Stay with
the trembling as long as possible and continue to breathe fully.

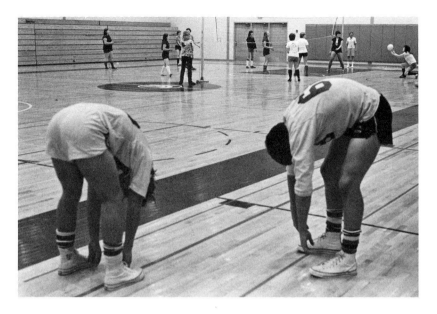

4.50. Hip bend. Use the yogic hip joint bend (illustrated in chapters 2 and 3) to relax the back muscles. Player on the left is bending from the waist; player on the right is bending from his back. Neither has learned the most effective way to release tension.

As you continue to practice this and other yogic exercises, you may become aware of tension and aches in other parts of the body. This is a good sign and indicates that body rigidity is being broken up. You can find a specific tension-releasing exercise for any area of the body in chapter 5. You should use these exercises liberally.

BASEBALL

Baseball is probably the most popular team sport in America. Early in the spring of each year, the bats, balls, and gloves are taken out in anticipation of spring training. From Little League and sandlot to the pros, the grand old game of baseball takes to the field.

As in other sports, the baseball player will benefit tremen-

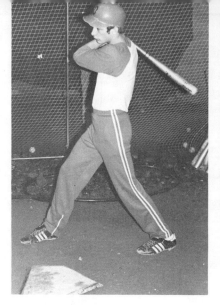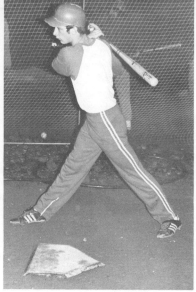

4.51, 4.52. Batting. Compare the correct swing (left) to the awkward swing on the right. The weight should remain on the back leg instead of being thrown forward.

dously from the regular practice of yogic breathing and balancing exercises described in chapters 1 and 3. The exercises that follow are specific applications of these basic principles, designed to refine your technique and performance.

BATTING

A good batter is a consistent hitter who combines balance with timing. Better balance can be mastered with repeated practice of the exercises in chapter 3, and every player is urged to spend as much time as possible with them. The following drill will help you transfer yogic balance and alignment to your action at the plate.

Work in an open space where you can swing a bat freely. Stand for a few minutes in the basic stance; then pick up a bat and assume the proper batting position—elbows off the body and hands back. Your breathing should be full and comfortable. Shift your weight to the back foot, with the weight falling into the ground along the outside foot and heel. Now slowly step forward 6 to 8 inches with the lead foot, as if you were about to swing at a ball. Imagine moving the sole of the foot, rather than the ankle or leg. Swing slowly and evenly, keeping the weight on the back foot and stepping forward from the sole of the lead foot. Notice how the hips come through without any effort.

THE CATCHER

The catcher demands special attention because of his unique crouching position. A collapsed crouching position can wear heavily on both the legs and the spine. On the other hand, a yogic crouch—the weight on the outside of the feet, whether the heels are off the ground or not—will not. The rib cage should be lifted with breath so the abdomen area will feel relaxed and spacious. Practice by moving from the fundamental stance to a crouching position while you do full yogic breathing.

Additional wear and tear can be avoided by learning how to rise from the crouch when you throw the ball. Again, move from the fundamental stance into the crouch. Now rise by applying pressure into the ground. The pressure starts at the feet, not the

4.53. The catcher. Bring foot forward as you rise, in a smooth motion with the throw.

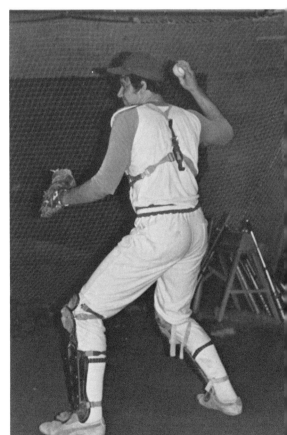

knees, which should feel as if they are moving down and back under the torso. (This will help take away the effort of lifting the body.) As you rise, the upper body should be erect. Practice the rise several times with full concentration on the movement. The idea is to let go of strain and effort so that you quickly and smoothly spring into the upright position by pressing into the ground.

The next step is to facilitate the transition from the crouched to the throwing position. Start raising your throwing hand and moving your foot forward to throw *as you rise*, as in illustration 4.53.

To develop the most efficient movement, think of lifting the sole of the foot off the ground rather than of lifting the leg. When you rise and prepare to throw in one smooth motion, you will discover that your movement will be quicker and your body more relaxed.

MODIFIED PLOUGH

This is a modification of a traditional yoga exercise that we have found to be particularly helpful for baseball players because it releases the muscles along the back of the legs and through the hips.

Work on a mat or rug and lie down on your back. Use a pillow to support your hips, and bring your feet straight back over your head. Your knees should be relaxed and your breathing full. Shortly after you begin the exercise, you should feel a trembling action in your legs and hips. Allow the trembling to increase and stay with the position for 15 minutes or longer.

Baseball players can also benefit from working with the exercises in the running and jogging section as well as the releasing exercises in the next chapter.

BASKETBALL

Every basketball player should take full advantage of his height. Yet, surprisingly, the posture of many players is so poor

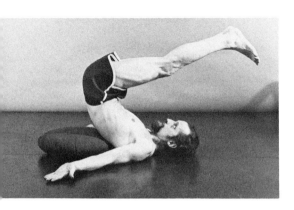

4.54. The modified plough. This relaxes muscles along the back of the legs and through the hips.

that they are losing a full inch or more. The reasons for this vary from person to person, but we have noticed that many players at one time were very uncomfortable about being so tall and had subconsciously drooped their shoulders and collapsed their rib cages in an effort to appear smaller. Also, the very real danger of hitting one's head on door frames and low ceilings contributes to the tall person's stoop.

Exercises in the chapters on basic yogic breathing and balance will elongate the body and bring it to its full height. These exercises, along with those in the running and jogging sections, should be practiced by every basketball player.

We designed the following exercise specifically for the basketball players we have worked with. It will help you to experience the full range of upper body motion as it gently stretches and releases muscles. You will get maximum benefit if you combine it with full yogic breathing.

SPACEWHEEL

There are two basic movements in this exercise, and they occur simultaneously—a twisting of the torso and legs and a swinging of the arms. The best way to describe this exercise, however, is to distinguish each movement separately. Happily, the exercise is much simpler to perform than it is to describe.

Part one

Stand with your knees relaxed and your feet about 12 inches apart. Slowly twist the torso as far to the right as you can, and then allow the feet to rotate so you are facing directly backward. Turn the right foot out until it has rotated about 90 degrees, or one quarter the way around an imaginary circle while you pivot on the ball of the left foot with the heel up and rotate it about 180 degrees so that it is pointed in the direction you are facing. Now, slowly rotate back and then all the way to the left. This time the left foot will be at an approximate right angle to the body while the right foot will be pointed in the direction you are facing. Vary the pace from slow to fast and practice rotating back and forth until the movement becomes smooth and comfortable.

Part two

Now face straight ahead and raise your hands straight above the top of your head with the fingers gently touching one another. Bring the arms down to the sides, as if they were mapping out large semicircles, and let the hands meet in front of the body. Immediately raise the hands together again, high over the head, and swing them down as you did before. The arm motion should be a smooth continuous swing of the hands. Practice at various speeds until the movement feels comfortable.

In the complete spacewheel, you will perform the torso twist and arm swing simultaneously. To give you some idea of the relative rhythms, you should complete about six arm swings in the time it takes to twist all the way around to one side. Continuing to twist at a slow pace, you will do approximately 24 swings for each *full* rotation. (Look at illustrations 4.55 to 4.60.) Breathe fully and get the sense of the body's opening and stretching as it pivots and swings through space. As you practice this exercise, you can get an even fuller turn and stretch; in a fuller spacewheel the feet will rotate further around.

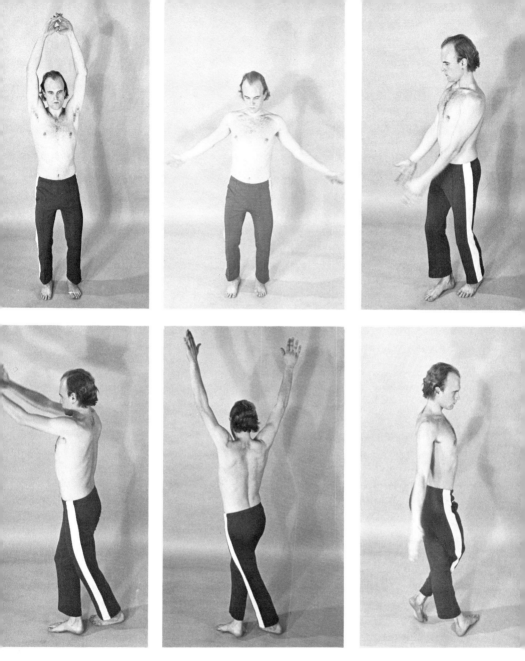

4.55.–4.60. The spacewheel. Here it is, step by step. It may be easier to work through the leg movements first and then the arm and torso movements. The purpose? To increase the full range of upper body motion on the basketball court.

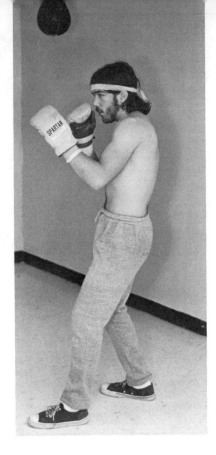

4.61. Using the ground. Shift from the outside of one foot to the outside of the other for maximized power and balance.

BOXING

The yogic principles for the boxer are designed to help develop a more relaxed technique with greater power and balance.

The secret to a powerful punch is the ability to transfer the maximum amount of energy from the whole body into the fist. The boxer's strength comes from the ground; therefore, a proper stance is exceptionally important. If, like many boxers, you assume your strength comes from your upper body and not from the ground, try jumping in the air and punching at the bag at the same time. This will illustrate how little power is in a punch when you are not using the ground.

USING THE GROUND

If you have mastered the fundamental yoga stance described

earlier in this book, you are well on your way to maximizing power and balance. Stand in this basic position, with the weight radiating down the outsides of your legs and feet, and then move into the regular boxing stance. Keep your knees slightly bent and feel the power of being firmly rooted by shifting your weight from the outside of one foot to the outside of the other.

The movement should come from pushing against the ground with your feet and not from the hips or knees. Move around and play with this motion by planting your feet in one position and then swaying from one foot to the other, keeping the weight on the outsides of the feet. Then move to another spot on the ground, and plant and sway again. You can do this until the body becomes familiar with the proper use of the ground. This will not build up a flat-footed style; it will help you to feel the

4.62. Move to another spot; plant and sway.

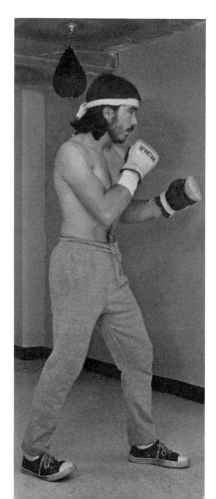

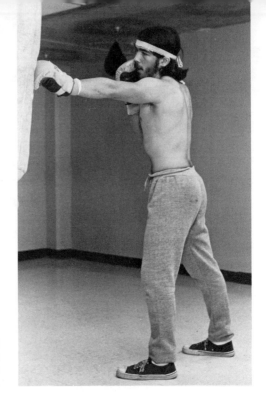

4.63. Jab from a relaxed position so that power comes from the ground, up through the body, and into the bag.

ground and know its importance in the development of true power.

Once you have a sense of the proper boxing stance, with the weight along the outsides of the feet, practice with a sparring bag. Hold your arms in the normal boxing pose, but try to get the sensation that they are relaxed in space and not being held up with any tension. The whole upper body should feel relaxed, and the breathing should be full and comfortable. Your buttocks should feel relaxed, and your weight should be concentrated on your heels. Now, jab the bag from this relaxed position. Can you sense that the power comes from the ground, up through the body, and into the bag?

Second in importance to being properly grounded is what is called a boxer's *style*. If you have watched Muhammad Ali, you have seen the open, more erect stance he uses. This is a completely different style from that of a crouching fighter. Ali's use of the ground and space is closer to the correct yogic method of motion and the proper use of the body's energy than is the classical, crouched style. If you are properly breathing and standing, you will discover how much more comfortable and effective the open style is. At first it may seem as if you are overexposing your body to the opponent, but the open, grounded body can more quickly handle a threat than the crouched, guarded body of the traditional fighter.

The boxer can benefit tremendously by doing deep yogic breathing between rounds in order to attain maximum recovery. The jogging and running exercises in this book will help the boxer develop breathing sufficiently so that proper breathing can be used both in training and in the ring. The exercises in the next chapter will be helpful in releasing tensions of the legs and upper body that are common to fighters.

THE BENCH

In most sports, athletes spend at least half their time waiting on the sidelines or on the bench before and during a game. This is especially true in such games as baseball, basketball, football, and hockey. This time could be extremely valuable for preparing the body for action, but it is an almost totally neglected opportunity for physical conditioning.

Free time during a game should be used to accomplish two things: relaxation and revitalization. On the field or on the bench, this is accomplished by yogic breathing and an aligned standing position.

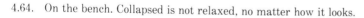
4.64.   On the bench. Collapsed is not relaxed, no matter how it looks.

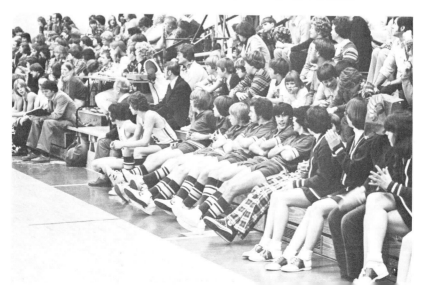

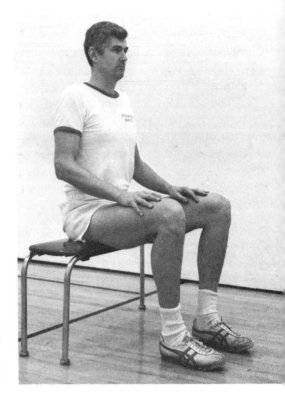

4.65. Sitting for vitality. Feet apart, spine straight but not rigid, neck straight, lower jaw loose, this player is gathering energy instead of wasting it.

On the bench, most athletes "relax" by collapsing or propping the body up in one way or another. This looks relaxed but in fact is not: A collapsed posture with the body out of alignment actually burns more energy than it appears to conserve and inhibits full and proper breathing.

SITTING FOR VITALITY

Start to practice this exercise in comfortable clothing. Sit on a bench or hard chair and place both feet firmly on the floor with the weight of the legs dropping into the ground along the outsides of the feet. Your feet should be your shoulders' width apart. Be aware of the seat beneath you, and make sure you are sitting on your "sit" bones and not on the small of your back.

Your hands can be placed comfortably on your thighs, and your spine should feel straight but not rigid. Bring in your chin so that the neck is straight and your head is centered above the shoulders. The lower jaw should feel loose and relaxed.

Now take a deep storage breath, filling the upper lungs and expanding the rib cage. The inhale should be so full that you feel the collarbone and shoulders lifting with the breath; the last portion of this deep storage breath should reach down into the abdominal area. Now do yogic breathing, as described in chapter 1, with a panting action and without losing the storage breath. Breathe like this for at least 10 minutes, and then allow the breathing to become slower and more comfortable. Should you lose some of the storage breath, be sure to replace it. While breathing, be aware of the body.

After you have learned how to sit and breathe properly, the next step is to move into action without losing the continuity of proper breathing. You should move from the bench to the field without a break in your awareness, breathing, or alignment.

From the sitting position, lift both feet slightly off the ground and then let them fall down hard. As they touch the ground, press down through the heels and the outsides of the feet, raising the torso straight up off the chair or bench. You should now be standing straight, but not rigid, in the basic stance. Repeat this motion while breathing, and soon you will be able to make the transition from sitting to standing without a loss of breath or attention.

If you are standing on the sidelines or on the field, you should evenly distribute your weight on both feet. The common stance for most people throws the weight of the body into one hip and leg. For the athlete, who must have ready energy, this position is disaster: It guarantees muscle fatigue. In football, when standing around, use the basic stance technique. The legs can then shake off tension and revitalize themselves.

All this may seem formal and unnatural at first, but, as you become familiar with basic yogic principles of true relaxation, you will be quite comfortable with proper body alignment. You will also be able to recognize poor postural habits. Then you will be using the time between actual play to your fullest advantage.

5

Fine tuning the athlete's body and mind

It is ironic that we have to work in order to relax and to practice in order to move naturally. But after years of improper use, we can't suddenly expect the body to align itself perfectly. Certain areas of the body will release rapidly while others will be more resistant to change; with regular practice and awareness, you will gradually arrive at a completely natural way of moving and using the body in sports.

If you have been working regularly with the basic breathing and balancing exercises presented in the first three chapters, you should already feel a change in your body—and possibly in your athletics, as well. The body should feel fuller, taller, and more spacious. On the other hand, you may still notice aches and pains that are hangovers from old injuries or are built-up emotional tensions. The exercises in this chapter are designed to further your progress by working through the entire body, from the mind to the toes.

We begin with some exercises for quieting the mind and heightening your awareness, since this practice will improve the effectiveness of every exercise you do. Yogis know that our ideas, attitudes, and emotions are incorporated in our bodies and influence our physical condition and posture. Therefore it is usually never enough simply to release tension in the muscles and joints. We also must shake off the rigid ideas and negative emotions that are partly responsible for our problems. Only when the mind is freed from rigidity and negativity and quieted from tensions can we experience an extended and profound state of release and relaxation.

Quieting the mind

Whether they are due to a losing streak in your play or an upset in your personal life, negative emotions such as depression, grief, and fear slow down activity. The upper body tends to slump, and the breathing becomes shallow. As a result, you experience a feeling of having less and less energy. Although the loss of energy seems real, the truth is that all the energy you need is always available. What happens in times of depression is that all this energy becomes short-circuited in a web of self-destructive thought and emotional activity.

Anger works in an equally destructive way, carrying rigidity and inflexibility throughout the body. The neck and jaw are particularly susceptible to this tension; frequently they become so tight it is difficult to breathe fully. Exercises that simply relieve tension may bring temporary relief, but by themselves they will not alleviate the harmful influence of the negative emotions.

The next time you become aware of a negative emotional state, apply the following principles to expand your awareness and release the negative energy.

1. Breathe with full yogic breaths and get the idea of sending the air into any areas of rigidity or collapse.

2. As you reach into these areas with the breath, allow the body to release through any movement or sound that may spontaneously arise.

3. Do not identify with the negative emotions and the thoughts that arise. When you do identify, thinking it is you instead of recognizing it as a psychological state you're passing through, you perpetuate the negative condition and it worsens. Try to see these emotions as the residue of past events. They need not exist now. Exorcise the negativity by allowing any sounds (moans, groans, laughter, shaking, or whatever) to leave the body with the exhale breath and vanish into the open space around you.

MEDITATION

Of course the best way to free yourself from negativity would be to let go of any negative emotion as soon as it arises. Unfortunately for most of us, this is practically impossible because we have almost no control over our thoughts, positive or negative.

At times the mind is like a grasshopper, randomly jumping from one object to another; it may seem to be moving along on whim and fancy. At other times the mind is like an animal trapped in quicksand, so overwhelmed with an idea or emotion that it cannot escape and think of anything else.

Yogis have known for a long time that negative emotions build up muscular tension and affect the entire circulatory system, as well as bring about a distracted state of mind that hinders performance. They also realize that a clear and quieted mind is essential to health. Thus they developed exercises, commonly called meditation practices, to still mental activity. The yogic healing breath and yogic healing walk that follow are meditation exercises for the beginner.

YOGIC HEALING BREATH

This exercise in breathing is designed to relieve physical and emotional tension through relaxation and awareness. It is an excellent way to begin any yogic exercise.

Sit in a chair with a straight back and hard seat. Your spine should be properly aligned without being rigid; your feet should be flat on the floor, in a line with your shoulders. Be sure you are sitting on your "sitting" bones and not your spine. Keep your chin in and your head centered. Place your hands on your thighs with the palms up. Breathe fully, without forcing the breath.

Focus your attention on your abdomen, about an inch below the navel, and be aware of the in-and-out action. Notice the abdomen filling up with air, and notice it emptying out the air. Keep your awareness on each rise and fall in the abdomen area. If you have difficulty noticing the expansion and contraction, place your hands on your abdomen and feel the movement.

The idea in this exercise is to sit in a relaxed way with your attention on only one thing: the expanding and contracting action of the abdomen. When a thought or idea comes up, simply note it and let it go. Keep your attention on the rising and falling action of the abdomen. If an emotion or physical sensation comes up, an itch or an idea, simply note it without doing anything. Don't scratch or get up.

As you observe thoughts bubbling up, watch for the instant when one thought falls away and another arises. It's possible to discover the gap or space between the two. If you can, attend to it; the gap or space will expand and the thought process will slow down and finally completely cease to cloud your clear, immediate experience of the moment.

Start by practicing the yogic healing breath for 15 minutes and gradually lengthen the time to half an hour. This is an excellent exercise first thing in the morning or before practicing yoga.

YOGIC HEALING WALK

As in the previous exercise, the idea here is to observe and quiet the mind. Practice in a space where you can take at least 25 to 50 steps without having to turn around (or walk in a circle, changing direction each time you arrive at the starting point). Start from the fundamental stance and slowly lift your right foot; move it forward, gently placing it down, and finally shift the weight onto it.

Just as you kept your awareness on the rising and falling of the abdomen in the previous exercise, here your awareness should be on the upward lift, forward movement, and gentle placement of the foot on the ground. Be aware of each phase of movement. Look straight ahead as you walk, and keep the arms relaxed and slightly extended from the sides of the body. When an emotion or idea arises, simply be aware of it; don't get involved. Turn your concentration to the slow action of the walk. Each time you run out of walking space (or complete your circle), note the intention to stop. Then stop, note the intention to turn around, and then turn around. Continue walking with full awareness of the movement in the opposite direction. Follow the directions for handling thought or sensations or emotions as stated in the healing breath section.

This exercise should be practiced for 15 minutes at first and gradually be extended to 30 minutes. An hour-long session that alternates 15-minute periods of the Yogic Healing Breath with the Yogic Healing Walk is highly recommended. When you end your exercise, try to keep your sense of relaxation and heightened awareness with you as you go about your daily activities.

Freeing the body

The following exercise should be done in a relaxed state of mind and with full attention. If possible, begin each session with 15 minutes of the yogic healing breath or walk; then work with the body. These exercises will not only bring greater flexibility to various joints, but they also will speed recovery to an injured part of the body. Go through the entire series of movements and then give greater attention to those areas of your body in greatest need of release or of most importance in your sport.

FREEING THE ANKLES

Lie on the floor with a hard pillow under your calves, with the heel and ankle joint of each leg suspended from the end of the pillow (about two inches off the ground). Direct your attention to your heels and the backs of your ankle joints; slowly bring your feet back toward the body and then slowly extend them as far forward as possible until your toes are pointing forward.

Continue this forward-and-backward stretch for at least 15 minutes. Be sure to keep your full attention on the ankles. If you practice long enough, you are sure to experience trembling and shaking, which signal releases in the muscles around the ankle joint.

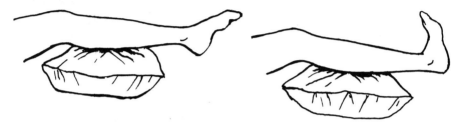

5.1.   Freeing the ankles. Slowly flex all the way down and back.

There are two other effective movements you can experiment with in the same position. Instead of moving the feet backward and forward, move them apart laterally at the ankle, as far out as they will go and then as far in as they will go, bringing the soles of the feet as close to facing one another as you can.

Again, practice for at least 15 minutes with full attention.

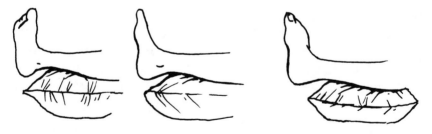

5.2.   Freeing the ankles. Move to the left and the right, bringing the soles as close together as you can.

Or, slowly rotate the feet in full circles, bringing them as far up, to the side, down, to the opposite side, and up again as you can. Rotate in both a clockwise and counterclockwise direction.

Remember, you are looking for a shaking and releasing action. Choose the movement that brings the most shaking and concentrate on it.

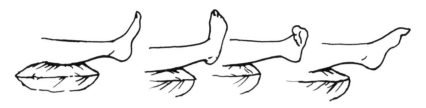

5.3. Freeing the ankles. Slowly rotate in full circles, clockwise and then counter-clockwise.

UNKNOTTING THE CALF

Tightly knotted calf muscles are common to many runners and athletes. They can be extremely painful, and by shortening the Achilles tendon, they also can adversely affect the flexibility of the foot and ankle and thereby increase the likelihood of sprains and injuries.

5.4, 5.5. Unknotting the calves. Slowly raise the heels, pressing the ground with the outside toes (left). Then slowly lower the heels.

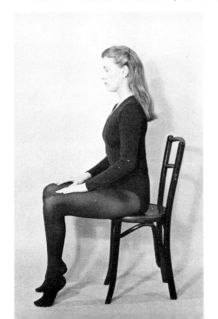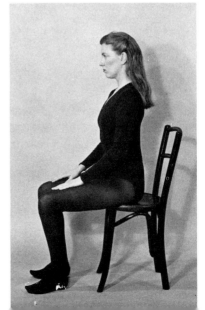

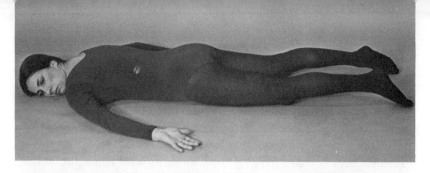

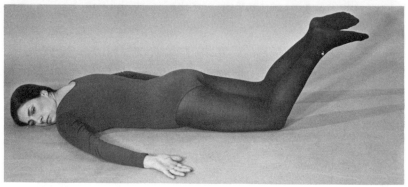

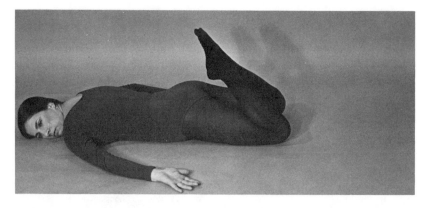

5.6.–5.8. Freeing the knees and thighs. Face down, arms out, slowly bring both feet toward the buttocks, then lower them to the floor.

Take off your shoes and sit in a chair with your feet about 6 inches apart, directly in front of you. Now press the ground down with the outside toes as you simultaneously lift the heels as high as possible. Still pressing into the ground with the outside toes, slowly lower the heels (5.4, 5.5).

Continue this raising and lowering motion, being sure the calf muscles stay as soft as possible. Note when the trembling begins, and allow the legs to shake up and down if they feel like it. Violent shaking is not uncommon with very tense calves. Allow the release to occur.

FREEING THE KNEES AND THIGHS

Lie on your stomach with your arms out to your sides, palms up. Bend the knees and slowly bring both feet all the way back toward the buttocks and down again to the floor, as in illustrations 5.6, 5.7, and 5.8. Repeat for at least 20 minutes.

FREEING THE PELVIC GIRDLE AND THIGHS

Muscular tension in the pelvic area can be particularly damaging to the body, because it throws out the entire posture of the upper body while it also cramps the space in the thighs and legs. Releasing the pelvic girdle makes a dramatic difference throughout the body.

Lie on your back with your knees bent and your feet flat on

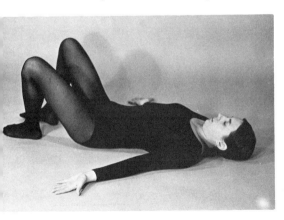

5.9, 5.10. Freeing the pelvic girdle and thighs. Arms out, knees bent, slowly roll feet outward and stretch legs apart; then roll feet and legs back together.

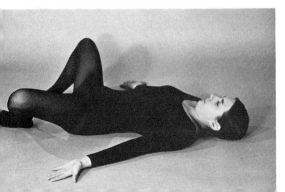

the floor, about 6 inches apart and about 10 inches from your buttocks. Take a full storage breath and be sure you continue to do yogic breathing throughout the exercises.

Extend your arms comfortably out from the body with your palms facing up and your fingers separated and extended. Without sliding your feet forward or backward, slowly separate your knees by rolling both feet out until your legs are as far down on each side as possible, without strain. Now slowly bring the knees together by rolling the feet back to the original position (5.9, 5.10).

Continue to open and close your legs in this manner for at least 15 minutes. In time, shaking will occur in the thighs and throughout the groin and pelvic area; it may even extend into the lower back. If you find one place in the movement where the

5.11, 5.12. Freeing the pelvic girdle and thighs. Feet angled on a chair or couch, open and close knees and thighs.

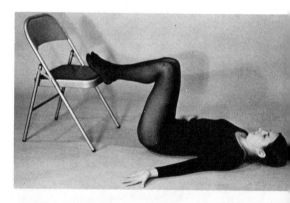

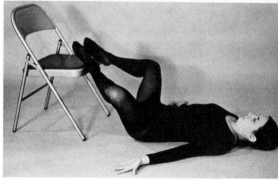

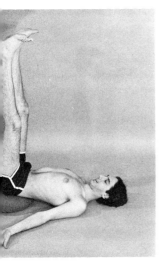 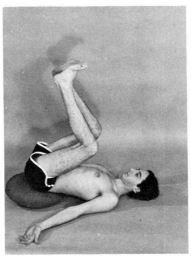 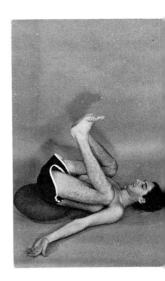

5.13–5.15. Freeing the pelvic girdle and thighs. Raise the feet and legs (left). Then slowly lower the knees to the chest, keeping feet together.

shaking is greatest, confine your motion to that area and allow the shaking to release tension.

Here's another variation of the exercise you should experiment with. Lie on your back, perhaps with several firm pillows under your buttocks. Place your feet on the seat of a chair or a couch so that your knees are bent at approximately the same angle as in the previous exercise, and repeat the same opening and closing movement in this upward angle position.

Here's a final exercise to bring release in the pelvic area. Place a pillow under your buttocks and raise the feet until the legs are perpendicular to the floor. Slowly bring the knees down toward the chest, as far as they will go without forcing them as in illustrations 5.13, 5.14, and 5.15.

Then slowly return to the original position with knees straight and legs and feet pointing straight up in the air. Repeat this movement for at least 20 minutes, allowing shaking to occur.

From the basic sensations you experience in these exercises, you may be able to invent some of your own that bring release to the pelvic area. Don't hesitate to experiment; do follow the

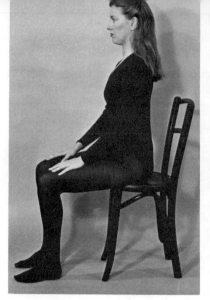
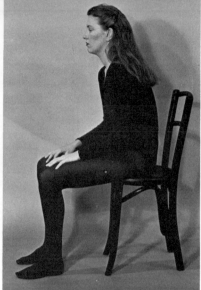

5.16–5.18. Freeing the lower back. Keeping shoulders in line with hips and head straight, curve spine out (top, right) and arch back forward (lower, right), simultaneously lifting the rib cage.

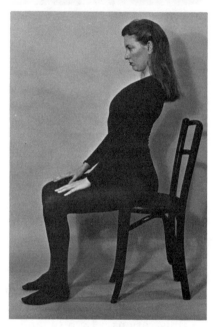

instincts of your body. Anything that brings shaking and trembling without strain will be valuable.

FREEING THE LOWER BACK

This is traditionally a trouble spot for many people. The

following exercise will help to strengthen the muscles of the lower back and to release tensions that distort a natural posture.

Sit forward on a hard chair, with the weight of your legs going into the ground through the outsides of the feet. Keep your feet about 6 to 8 inches apart and breathe deeply. Throughout this exercise, the shoulders should be directly above the hips.

With the exhale, drop the rib cage down toward the hips, curving the spine out. On the inhale, arch your back forward and lift the rib cage. Repeat this collapsing and arching motion, slowly in the beginning and then varying the pace until you find the greatest trembling and releasing action. Keep your head

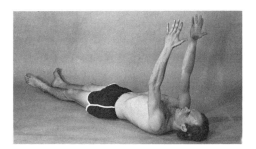

5.19–5.21. Freeing the arms and shoulders. Raise hands and arms and let the weight drop through the shoulders and into the ground. Then slowly lower hands to the side, until they form a "T" with the body.

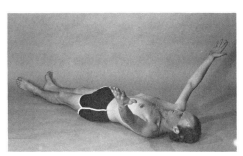

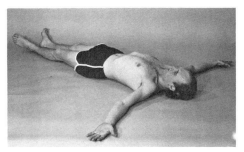

straight throughout the exercise. As you continue, you will be able to feel trembling all the way up through the upper back and neck and down through the thighs and lower leg.

FREEING THE ARMS AND SHOULDERS

Lie on your back and raise your hands until they are perpendicular to the floor, with the palms facing one another about 6 inches apart and elbows straight but not tense. Let the weight of the arm drop through the shoulder and into the ground. Now, slowly lower the hands to the sides, until they touch the ground and form a "T" with the body. Then slowly raise the hands, bringing them up until the palms meet.

5.22–5.24. Freeing the arms and shoulders. Arms outstretched, place hands behind the head, palms down. Raise hands over the head and then lower them, as close as possible to the side of the body.

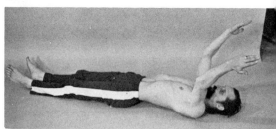

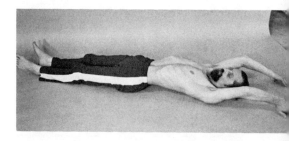

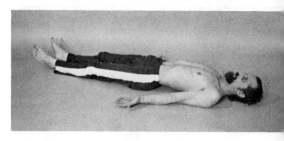

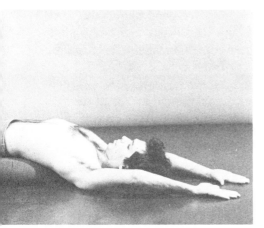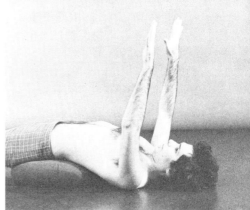

5.25, 5.26. Freeing the arms and shoulders. Stretch hands out behind the head, palms up (left). Slowly raise until they are directly over the body.

Allow full trembling to occur in the arms and across the chest. Repeat this motion and then try the following two variations.

• Lie on your back and place your hands behind your head, arms outstretched and palms down. Bring the hands up and over the head and all the way down to the ground, as close to the side of the body as possible, and then return the hands to their original position behind the head. Repeat this motion slowly.

• Place a pillow under the small of your back. Stretch your hands out behind your head, with the palms facing up. Slowly raise your outstretched hands and arms up until they are directly over the body and perpendicular to the floor (5.25, 5.26).

Then lower the hands and repeat the up-and-down motion until trembling occurs; then continue to allow this for at least 5 to 10 minutes.

FREEING THE CHEST AND UPPER BACK

This simple exercise is remarkably effective in freeing the chest and upper back areas.

Lie on your back and place your outstretched hands and arms behind your head with the palms up. Raise your arms and hands about 6 inches off the floor and rotate them along the floor, all the way down until the hands meet the thighs.

Without raising or lowering the hands and arms, rotate them back again behind the head. Continue this motion for at least 15 minutes.

FREEING THE ELBOW

Lie on your back with your hands and arms straight up,

5.27–5.29. Freeing the chest and upper back. Hands above the body, palms up, raise about 6 inches off the floor and move to shoulder height (center) and continue to the thighs.

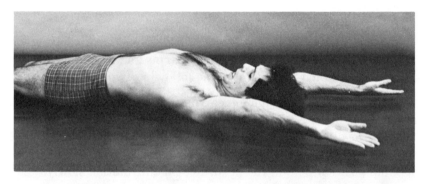

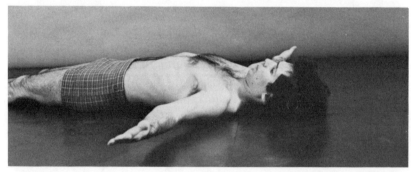

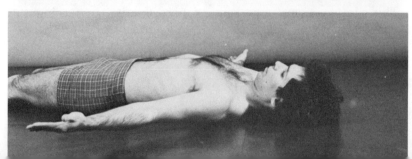

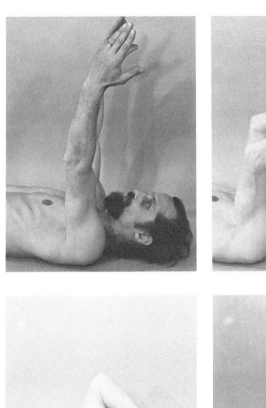
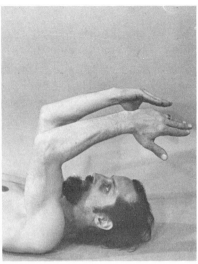
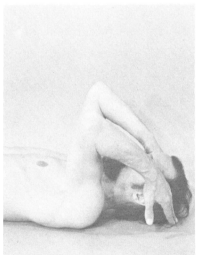
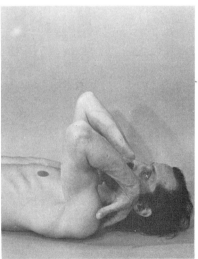

5.30–5.33.   Freeing the elbow. Hands up, palms backward, slowly lower fingers until they touch the ground just behind your head (lower left). Then slowly slide the fingers forward to touch the shoulders.

perpendicular to the floor. Face the palms backward, with your fingers separated and extended. Now slowly bring your fingers down until they touch the ground just behind the head; then slowly slide the fingers forward until the palm touches the shoulders. Slide the fingers back and raise the hand to its original upright position.

During the movement the upper arms should move as little as

5.34–5.36. Freeing the elbow. From the starting position (top), bring hands off the floor toward shoulder (center), without raising upper arm. Then move arms slowly back to original position.

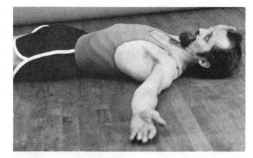

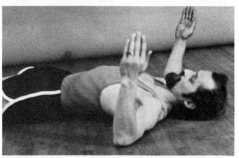

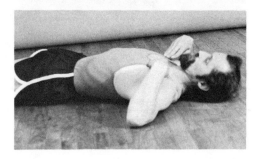

possible. You will experience shaking in the lower arm, biceps and into the shoulder.

In a variation of this exercise, place your arms on the ground at right angles to the body, again with the fingers outstretched and the palms facing upward. Slowly arc the palm toward the shoulder without raising the arm.

As you continue these exercises, you may find that the shaking shifts the lower arm position; allow the arms to fly out or shake in any direction they feel like.

FREEING THE NECK

Sit in a hard chair or stand with your spine straight. Take a full storage breath and start deep yogic breathing. Eyes closed or looking straight ahead, tilt your head down toward your right shoulder, keeping the right ear in line with the shoulder joint (5.37).

Then slowly move the head back and forth until you feel the

5.37.   Freeing the neck. Begin deep yogic breathing. Tilt head toward right shoulder, keeping right ear in line with the shoulder joint. Slowly rotate head from side to side.

5.38.   At the strongest stretch (or most painful spot), slowly rotate head upward, without lifting the neck away from the shoulder.

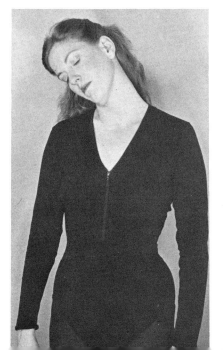
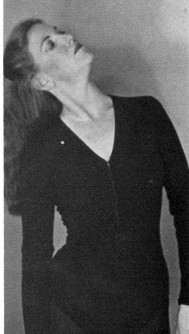

greatest stretch and pull along the left side of the neck without straining. When you have found the strongest stretch (possibly the most painful spot), slowly rotate your head upward, without lifting the neck away from the shoulder (illustration 5.38).

The head will move as if the eyes were following the trajectory of an object that rises from the floor on your right side to the ceiling just above the left shoulder. Repeat the same motion with your head tilted down toward your left shoulder.

FREEING THE JAW, THROAT, AND FACE

If you are able, sit on your heels with the front of your feet flat on the floor. (If this position is too painful, sit in a chair.)

Open your mouth as wide as possible in all directions and extend your tongue, stretching it from the base, as far and as wide as you can.

Get the feeling of gently stretching the back of the throat at the same time. Take a full storage breath and pant. If your mouth gets too dry, close it for a few seconds and then resume the exercise. If any sounds come out as you pant, let them. If you wish, you may massage any sore areas in the jaw while doing this exercise.

5.39. Freeing the jaw, throat, and face. Open as wide as possible and pant.

5.40. Freeing the jaw, throat, and face.

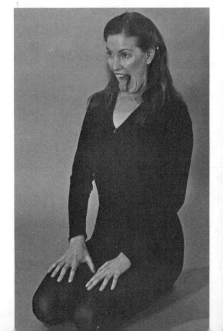
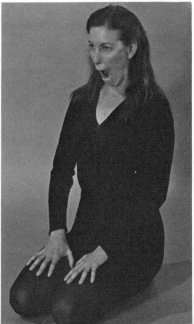

Here's another exercise that will help to relax the jaw and face. Open your mouth and cover your upper and lower teeth with your lips. Get the feeling of pulling your teeth back with your lips. Raise your eyebrows and, without tilting your head, look as far up as possible. Take a storage breath and pant.

Summary

When yoga is part of the active life of the athlete, the body gradually opens and relaxes, bringing about a growing awareness of movement, of the rising and passing away of body sensations, of thoughts and emotions.

The yogic athlete allows his or her body to perform without becoming identified with its successes and failures. If the athlete believes in being the possessor of movement, sensation, thought, or emotion, he or she darkens and clouds the open experience of space and motion. When ownership is claimed ("I did it"), the athlete becomes rigid and inflexible. A rigid attitude and posture may work for a while, but when circumstances change, the rigid athlete is unable to adapt and becomes confused because he or she no longer feels able to control the situation.

It's as if the athlete were a juggler in an open field: The rhythm is perfect and juggled balls make perfect arcs as they pass from one hand to the other. But suddenly the wind changes, and the path of the balls is altered. The rigid athlete will become paranoid and wonder what went wrong when the balls fail to fall into his or her hands.

The yogic athlete, on the other hand, is open to the environment and is one with it; he or she instinctively adapts to the change in wind. The yogic athlete does not try to control the wind but instead adjusts movement to it.

In this book we have presented you with a series of exercises to release tensions, bring about a natural alignment, and open your awareness. As you continue to combine yoga with your sport you will gradually come to master the field you play on— and your game will continually improve with experience.

Index